The Psychiatric Interview

By HARRY STACK SULLIVAN, M.D.

CLINICAL STUDIES IN PSYCHIATRY

CONCEPTIONS OF MODERN PSYCHIATRY

THE FUSION OF PSYCHIATRY AND SOCIAL SCIENCE

THE INTERPERSONAL THEORY OF PSYCHIATRY

PERSONAL PSYCHOPATHOLOGY

THE PSYCHIATRIC INTERVIEW

SCHIZOPHRENIA AS A HUMAN PROCESS

Prepared under the auspices of

THE WILLIAM ALANSON WHITE PSYCHIATRIC FOUNDATION
COMMITTEE ON PUBLICATION OF SULLIVAN'S WRITINGS

Mabel Blake Cohen, M.D.   Dexter M. Bullard, M.D.
David McK. Rioch, M.D.   Janet MacK. Rioch, M.D.
Clara Thompson, M.D.
Helen Swick Perry, *Editorial Consultant*

W. W. NORTON & COMPANY

New York · London

HARRY STACK SULLIVAN, M.D.

THE
Psychiatric
Interview

Edited by
HELEN SWICK PERRY *and* MARY LADD GAWEL
With an Introduction by OTTO ALLEN WILL, M.D.

W · W · NORTON & COMPANY
New York · London

Prepared under the auspices of

THE WILLIAM ALANSON WHITE PSYCHIATRIC FOUNDATION
COMMITTEE ON PUBLICATION OF SULLIVAN'S WRITINGS
Mabel Blake Cohen, M.D.   Dexter M. Bullard, M.D.
David McK. Rioch, M.D.   Otto Allen Will, M.D.

First published in the Norton Library 1970

ISBN 0-393-00506-2

Published simultaneously in Canada by
Penguin Books Canada Ltd,
2801 John Street, Markham, Ontario L3R 1B4.

W. W. Norton & Company, Inc. is also the publisher of the
works of Erik H. Erikson, Otto Fenichel, Karen Horney, Harry Stack
Sullivan, and The Standard Edition of the Complete Psychological
Works of Sigmund Freud.

W. W. Norton & Company, Inc., 500 Fifth Avenue,
New York, N.Y. 10110
W. W. Norton & Company Ltd. 37 Great Russell Street,
London WC1B 3NU

PRINTED IN THE UNITED STATES OF AMERICA
1 2 3 4 5 6 7 8 9 0

Contents

Reissued in Sullivan's *Psychology, a procedure whose purpose . . .
ful in the preparation of the first of these books.

Editors' Preface

THIS is the second of the posthumous books of Harry Stack Sullivan prepared under the auspices of the William Alanson White Psychiatric Foundation, Sullivan's literary executor. This book is based on two lecture series which Sullivan gave, in 1944 and again in 1945, under the title of *The Psychiatric Interview*. These lectures were given in the Washington School of Psychiatry, which is the training institution of the Foundation. While the lectures were directed primarily toward psychiatrists, Sullivan also meant them for all those who engage in dynamic interviewing. The lectures were recorded, and this book is based both on these recordings and on two Notebooks, one for each year, which Sullivan used as a guide in presenting his lectures. In general, Sullivan's own scheme of organization of the material, as he refined it in the second year, has been followed, and the best material from each year has been selected to cover the various topics. This has been supplemented by material drawn from three lectures on psychiatric interviewing which Sullivan included in a more general and theoretical lecture series in 1946–47. Thus this book endeavors to present all of the best of Sullivan on this topic and at the same time not to depart radically from Sullivan's organization of an approach to this topic.

Insofar as possible, Sullivan's language has been left intact. However, repetitions and digressions more appropriate to the lecture room than to the printed page have been omitted or footnoted, and obscurities have been clarified by reference to Sullivan's Notebooks, to what he said on the same points at other times, and by listening to the recordings themselves for the emphasis and meaning of sentences as spoken. The headings and subheadings in the book are mainly derived from the headings in Sullivan's Notebooks, a procedure which proved useful in the preparation of the first of these books.

Much of the material in the first two chapters of this book appeared first in the journal *Psychiatry* [(1951) 14:361–373 and (1952) 15:127–141]. In organizing this into book form, it has been necessary to shift some of the material and to make other minor modifications incident to the making of a book.

In presenting this book to the public, the Foundation wishes to make special mention of the contribution of Otto Allen Will, M.D., to the work on the clinical papers in general and this book in particular. Shortly after Sullivan's death, Dr. Will became interested in the possibility of organizing all of the various clinical lecture series into books. He began to put some of the various clinical lectures into readable form so that the richness of the material could be more easily recognized. His voluntary assumption of this role has played no small part in the Foundation's program for publishing this series of books. The selection and the preliminary assessment of the material in this book was done by Dr. Will, and he has acted as medical consultant in all phases.

In the preparation of this book we are particularly indebted to Philip A. Holman, a staff member of the journal *Psychiatry*, who has helped extensively in the editing and at various stages of the preparation of the book. For the typing of the final manuscript and the proofreading we wish to express our gratitude to Marguerite A. Martinelli.

Finally, we would like to pay tribute to the friends of the Foundation—students and colleagues of Sullivan's, for the most part—who continue to give financial support and encouragement to the whole project.

HELEN SWICK PERRY
MARY LADD GAWEL

Introduction

IN THIS book psychiatry is defined as the field of the study of interpersonal relations, emphasis being placed on the interaction of the participants in a social situation, rather than being centered exclusively on the supposedly private economy of either one of those participants. The psychiatric interview is a special instance of interpersonal relations, and the term, as used here, does not refer exclusively to the meeting of a psychiatrist and his patient. The interview is characterized by the coming together of two people, one recognized as an expert in interpersonal relations, the other known as the client, interviewee, or patient, who expects to derive some benefit from a serious discussion of his needs with this expert. The situation is designed to make clear certain characteristic patterns of the client's living with the prospect that such elucidation will prove useful to him.

The term psychiatric as used here simply indicates that the interview is considered to be an interpersonal phenomenon, and that the data for its study and comprehension are to be derived from the observation of what goes on between the participants—or, to phrase it in another way, from an observation of the field of their interaction. Also implied in the term is the concept that patterns of living are to be clarified and that in that process benefit may accrue to the client. Interview situations in which the goal is the obtaining of factual data from the interviewee—as in the presenting of a questionnaire —and in which subsequent benefit to the interviewee is of little or no importance, are not by this definition "psychiatric."

Thus the term psychiatric interview, as used in this book, has broad implications, and the discussion of it presented here is practically related not only to the psychiatrist and his patient, but to the interviewer and interviewee in a wide variety of situations. The term interview does not apply to a certain fixed period of time, but rather to a course of interpersonal events which may be encompassed to some degree in a single conference of sixty or ninety minutes' duration, or developed to a greater extent during the course of several meetings, or elaborated in the many sessions of intensive psychotherapy. Contained in a single psychiatric interview are the essential characteristics and movements of the more prolonged therapy. So it is that much of what is discussed here in terms of the interview has application to the entire course of a psychotherapeutic endeavor.

We often speak of the "art" of this or that—the art of salesmanship, of medicine, of living, of interviewing. Used in this way the term art may indicate that an important part of the profession or task is an interpersonal relationship, the skillful handling of which plays a large part in the success or failure of the enterprise. The word also suggests that the particulars of the relationship are not subject to observation and description; they are "intuitive," "subjective," or "personal," and likely to be damaged in some way by close scrutiny, or they are "insignificant" and "unscientific," and unsuited for objective study. Thus, to speak of the art of interviewing may imply that the processes in that interaction are not observable, and that for reasons not entirely clear, the situation might best flourish in an atmosphere of privacy.

Sullivan thought that the scientific method could be applied to study of the interpersonal field, and that patterns of action in the interview could be identified, observed, and defined in a manner that would move the entire process to some extent away from the obscurity of an art and toward the clarity of a science. He made some progress in this direction by paying considerable attention to the nonverbal components of the situation—tone of voice, patterning of speech, facial expression, bodily gesture, and so on—the ways by which so much of meaning is transmitted between people, and the observation of which is often indiscriminately labeled by some such term as intuition. Sullivan also observed that the processes in the interview are kept obscure by the mutual anxiety of the participants. Thus it is easier for the patient to think of his relationship to the therapist as puzzling, irritating, frustrating, unsatisfactory, or even wonderful, than to recognize the anxiety which has led to his puzzlement, irritation, wonderment, and so on. The therapist, likewise, may find it more comforting and less disturbing—although hardly more profitable—to consider his role in the interview as an artistic performance not subject to observation, thus avoiding a study of the interactions with his patient in which his own anxiety plays a significant part.

In the lectures from which this book originated, Sullivan was formulating his thinking concerning a theory of interpersonal relationships as applied to the special instance of the interview. A portion of the lecture time was spent in group discussion, the approach being one of inquiry, of formulating questions, and of suggesting approaches to the study of human behavior, rather than one of attempting to discover definite "answers" to alleged "problems." In later years this process or operational approach was further developed by Sullivan in a series of seminars concerned with interviewing. These were lively meetings in which students presented case material, discussion was encouraged, and the business of psychiatry as demonstrated in the group interaction was seen to be very much a matter of interpersonal relatedness. Except for notes made by students, there are no records of these seminars, and they are not reflected in this book.

Although the coming together of two people for the purpose of developing a meaningful exchange of ideas directed toward their mutual enlightenment is a fundamental characteristic of the interview, such a meeting is complicated by the disjunctive force of the anxiety experienced by both participants. The psychiatrist and the patient—the interviewer and the interviewee—are motivated to meet with each other by certain obvious considerations. The psychiatrist looks upon the meeting as a way of practicing his profession, and of earning his living. The patient comes in order to learn more of certain characteristics of his behavior which he finds to be in some ways a handicap, with the prospect of altering these to his greater satisfaction. Despite such motivations, which would seem to favor the rapid progress of communication, an outstanding feature of interviews is the fact that the patient will not find it simple to present his case, will frequently engage in evasions, the subtleties of which he may be unaware of, and may wish to withdraw from the situation before much benefit has been obtained. The psychiatrist may find his work interfered with by his own anger, boredom, inattention, and other responses which are seemingly inappropriate to the expert in this specialty. Thus both psychiatrist and patient, while strongly motivated to meet, are also driven by anxiety to withdraw from each other. This interplay of movements—multiple variations of advance and retreat—is characteristic of the field of the interview. These operations on the part of both psychiatrist and patient are inevitable accompaniments of an interview and therefore cannot reasonably be looked upon as cause for rejoicing or lamentation. Because of their display the patient need not be labeled as difficult or uncooperative, nor the psychiatrist as incompetent. Although the psychiatrist is expected to be alert to these subtle interactions, it is not likely that he will immediately identify all of them. The goal of interviewing is not to do away with these movements, but to recognize them, explore their origins, and come to an understanding of their significance in the current situation. It is with such relationships of forces in a social field that the present book is concerned.

There is nothing extraordinary in the concept that the participants in an interview may experience emotions which promote their mutual withdrawal. Although the experience of anxiety is always unpleasant, there is little likelihood in our world that we can avoid it at all times, despite our great capacities for developing remarkably effective patterns of behavior as forms of defense. If early acquaintance with anxiety has been markedly painful, he who has endured this will be cautious in his dealings with people, and loath to expose himself to relationships which may threaten his feeling of security. Such a one may not welcome becoming either a psychiatrist or a patient—the personal contacts which are an ingredient of either role may seem too painful to risk. Nevertheless, without the experience of anxiety one would not become a patient; and without such experience it is not likely that one would be so preoccupied with the subtleties of human performance as to become a psychiatrist.

For the psychiatrist his experience of anxiety can be put to good use in his dealings with his patients, as well as with others. For such experiences to be forged into a useful therapeutic tool they must be identified, brought into awareness, their origins and modes of expression understood, and their reality accepted as part of life without fear or shame. All this is simply a part of the business of being a competent psychiatrist and interviewer as these terms are used here.

Sullivan spent some time at St. Elizabeths Hospital in Washington, D. C., where he worked in association with William Alanson White, and had the opportunity of observing large numbers of patients diagnosed as schizophrenic. He then moved to Sheppard and Enoch Pratt Hospital in Maryland, where he passed several years in investigating the difficulties of acutely disturbed schizophrenic patients in a small hospital unit. During this period, Sullivan was studying the difficulties that people have in "making sense" with each other, in finding out what the other fellow "means." In doing this he came to an observing of the interaction of forces in a social field, and began to develop a method of thinking increasingly congenial with the concepts of the modern physical sciences, and with the trend of the social sciences. He was moving in the direction of the so-called operational approach to the study of communication.

In his work with schizophrenic patients Sullivan observed that they often used language more as a means of defense than of communication; their speech served to keep people at a distance, thus protecting an already low self-esteem. One who has experienced a great deal of anxiety in contacts with others tends to withdraw from those others. He may do this by physical avoidance, by "keeping his thoughts to himself," or by speaking in such a fashion that his listeners are bored, irritated, puzzled, call him "crazy," and in turn withdraw from him. All of this is not "conscious" or planned, but is a complicated response to anxiety; and the end result is very successful avoidance of people.

Following the period at Sheppard, Sullivan spent some time in working with those who are known as obsessional. Although their behavior was more conventional and socially acceptable than that of many schizophrenic people, the obsessional use of language could be comprehended as another elaborate defense against the decrease of self-esteem at the hands of another person, and the accompanying experience of anxiety. Certain aspects of human living in our culture were becoming increasingly clear. It was evident that anxiety was a common experience, that it had its origins in the relationships of people with one another, and that in response to it, defensive patterns, or security operations, were developed which served to isolate people and keep them at some distance from each other. In certain exaggerated form these patterns were known as symptoms and indicators of "mental disease." Psychiatric patients were being understood as essentially no different from other humans, and as but striking examples of the common human experience—namely, that from people can come not only great good—but also great harm. This most children learn early in their lives; they learn that they cannot exist without human contact, and they also learn that some of that contact is dangerous in its arousal of anxiety—as well as in other ways. Experience that leads one to emphasize the dangerous aspects of human contact, and to erect great barriers against these, is the background of those recognized as mentally disordered and of many another whose difficulties may be concealed by a conventional façade.

As he came to a greater understanding of the general destructive effects of the experience of anxiety, its commonness in everyday life, and the intimate relationship between what is called normal and abnormal living, Sullivan shifted his interests to teaching and to the furthering of the collaborative efforts of workers in the various fields of human relations. If the psychiatric patient was not a peculiar form of human mutation, or other expression of biological disaster, but was to a large extent a reflection of group living which directed the patterning of his behavior, just as it directed that of successful and normal people, then the role of the psychiatrist must change. Biological wreckage might be isolated and supervised in institutions, and scatterings of human deviants be treated by clinicians of a medical specialty. But as the interest of the psychiatrist widened, keeping pace with the newer concept of his patient as at least a partial expression of the social group, it became increasingly evident that psychiatric problems were hardly to be solved by the creation of large numbers of practitioners, however skilled, to minister to those who might conceivably benefit from their efforts.

It was a realization of something like this that led Sullivan to turn his attention from the details of dealing with anxiety in individual therapy to the problems concerned with the diminishing of anxiety—or tension—as it appeared in groups. From what he had learned in his study of the person in terms of the social setting, he came to a greater recognition of the importance of the social structure in relation to mental health and mental disorder. In 1948, the year before his death, he was active in forming the World Federation for Mental Health, and in serving as a participant in the UNESCO Tensions Project, established by the United Nations to study tensions affecting international understanding. In developing greater comprehension of the intimate relationship existing between the socially productive person and the emotionally disordered and less productive one, Sullivan came to look upon anxiety as a destructive commonplace in human living, as the motor of much group tension, and as a force of such significance in its effects that it should be dealt with by group and public-health measures. Preventive psychiatry and the application of psychiatric knowledge to other fields of study seemed to him of greater urgency than an exclusive preoccupation with individual therapy. In this thinking he was in the medical tradition. Few practitioners would relish treating tubercular patients without the backing of the public-health measures which are so effective in reducing the incidence of that disorder. If it is once clearly understood that a goodly number of the emotionally disordered are a reflection of their life experiences, and if it is also understood that few people even remotely approach any full realization of their potentialities, and that such wastage of human potential is practically expensive and destructive to the larger social group, serious attention might be paid to efforts directed at the prevention of such loss. For the psychiatrist the task is, at least, the increased clarification of the difficulties as he sees them in his patients, and the relating of those difficulties to the broader social scene, with an accompanying promotion of a wider recognition of those relationships.

Throughout his career Sullivan was concerned with problems of communication as these were demonstrated in a variety of situations—in numbers of patients in large hospital wards, in the obscure behavior of schizophrenic patients observed in close personal contact, in the more conventional life of the obsessional person, and in the interaction of groups, large and small. This book on the interview, based on lectures given in 1944 and 1945, is concerned with the phenomena that interfere with the freedom of communication, as they are revealed in the special instance of two people sitting down together for a supposedly common purpose—improving the living of one of them. No patient—and few people under any classification—come into the presence of another without considerable caution and some expectation of rebuff. The understanding of such blocks to communication, reflecting underlying anxiety and anticipation of hurt from another human, is a major goal of the interview. The interview itself may be looked upon as a miniature of all communicative processes, containing within it the essential qualities of all human relationships, and much data relevant to the getting along of people in any social setting.

It should be clear that this book does not present a definite schematization of just what the interviewer should do in conducting the interview. It is not intended as an outline guide for action, but rather as a provocative succession of ideas which may prove stimulating to the thinking of anyone who conducts an interview. Many of us, doctors, nurses, and others, have been brought up in the tradition of identifying problems and then doing something about them; as practical people we want to deal with a clear statement of a difficulty and a prescription for action. We want to see a beginning, a solution, and an end to a situation. If we could only be told that a patient's trouble arises at point A, that it can be defined as disease B, and that it can be relieved by the application of remedy C, through the use of technique D, we would feel as if we were getting somewhere. This book does not give such answers.

Sullivan was trying to make some formulation of a process, by which I mean an always progressing, never stable movement of interactions taking place between people. This dynamic interplay of forces in a social field is in constant motion even though the outward behavior of the participants suggests that an equilibrium exists. Such an equilibrium is dynamic in character, the relationship being maintained by the ever-shifting patterns of behavior of the parties involved in the field. The psychotherapeutic process—and the psychiatric interview seen as a segment of that process—may be looked upon in this operational manner, in which the person observed can be comprehended only in terms of his relationship to others who influence him in his "life space," or field of living, and in terms of the behavior of the observer—the therapist or interviewer—who is, of necessity, a part of that field. In this sense the study of the interview becomes a study of the process or the interaction which results from the presence of the participants in that field. From this study certain rather accurate inferences may be drawn as to the past experience of those participants as reflected in the current action. Questions and answers about such a field must then be what is often referred to as "open-ended" —that is, they cannot be conclusive, final, and in all ways precise. They *can* be suggestive, provocative, and useful in guiding further inquiry as one participates in and moves along with the process under study. The attempt to deal in fixed quantities

—raising questions as to 'Just what do I say here?', 'Just what does the patient mean when he says that?'—presents a static and somewhat unreal picture of the interview. 'What I say' and 'what the patient means' can be determined only in terms of the total context, and that context itself is not static. Thus in his consideration of the interview Sullivan reflects a movement in his own thinking toward an operational, field approach to the study of psychiatry, and his writing can be understood best when this developing point of view is kept in mind.

In working with schizophrenic patients, Sullivan found that the technique of so-called free association did not always yield great profit. The mute patient did not respond, the paranoid patient tended to repeat his paranoid stereotypes, and the patient who was near panic often came nearer to panic, engaging in great displays of "crazy" behavior which frequently effectively interrupted the relationship. The hebephrenic patient was usually not responsive to any suggestion to speak freely and easily. The obsessional person might speak at great length, but often with little apparent relevance to anything that might seriously constitute a problem in his living. The manic patient associated with all too great a show of freedom, and the depressed person withdrew even more when asked to relax and talk freely.

In this book Sullivan is not speaking "in favor of" an interview which is entirely directed by the therapist, and he is not speaking "against" the uncensored expression of the free flow of ideas. He is, however, opposed to the casual prescription of courses of action without there being some idea of how such action is to be effected. I recall that some years ago, when engaged in the more general practice of medicine, I advised a certain patient with high blood pressure to "take it easy." This gentleman was very polite, thanked me for my advice, and departed. Later, at my leisure, I was able to ponder on how this man, who supported a wife and three children by his labors in driving a dump truck, might apply my prescription. I decided that the prescription was not suited to the case, or that I should have devoted more attention to discovering how practical use might be made of it.

So for Sullivan and the matter of free association. He thought that the concept was excellent, but saw that the reasons for the difficulties of its application are intimately related to communication in the interview. To speak freely and without censorship implies a very low level of anxiety, a condition which rarely exists in the interview situation, unless the anxiety is covered by defensive maneuvers which in themselves are not useful expressions of free association. The questions raised by Sullivan are simply, 'How do you get people to associate freely?', and 'If there is trouble doing this, what is the nature of the trouble, and what can be done about it?' The very raising of such questions may be productive in improving the communication.

In these lectures Sullivan does not discuss countertransference as such, but he does place great emphasis on the role of the physician or interviewer. An important aspect of this role is the fact that one's observations of another may be considerably influenced by unrecognized anxieties arising from previous relationships with people. Such distortions we call transference or countertransference, depending on their reference to the patient or to the therapist. In Sullivan's thinking there is no situation in which the interviewer is a "neutral" figure in the therapeutic field; he is inevitably a participant, and the field of social action is altered by his presence. Thus the therapist can never observe his patient *acting-as-if-I-weren't-here-and-he'd-never-met-me*, but can see him only *acting-in-terms-of-his-past-and-including-me-also*. With this in mind it is evident that the removing of transference distortions does not do away with the fact that the social field is composed of the participants as real people plus the ways in which each experiences this current "reality" as a reflection of his previous experiences in living.

Sullivan had no great confidence in the accuracy of anyone's recall in reproducing either the content of an interview or its vocal and gestural accompaniments. Yet he thought that the taking of notes during an interview interfered with the exchange of ideas, and for a time was of the opinion that recording machines might unfavorably disturb the field. However, he was very much interested in the making of detailed observa-

XX   THE PSYCHIATRIC INTERVIEW

tions of the nonverbal aspects of communication, and in the later years of his life he used a recording machine during some of his hours of therapy, listening back to such recordings in an attempt to learn more clearly "what had gone on." He also listened to recordings of colleagues' work with their patients and hoped that in this way he would be able to increase his effectiveness as a consultant.

In 1948 Sullivan was instrumental in getting under way a project in which the entire course of therapy with three patients (each with a different therapist) was recorded, and subjected to careful review by the therapists and consultants. In this way there was a movement in the direction of subjecting the work of the therapist to detailed scrutiny, thus getting a closer look at what is so casually spoken of as the "therapeutic operation."

At present the recording of interviews and their study are increasingly commonplace. The next step—which has already been taken by some, and was proposed by Sullivan [1] in the late 1920's—is the photographing of interview sessions, with the goal of obtaining a good look at the nonverbal gestural components of communication. In doing this we may come to a greater understanding of many things which in this book are but suggested, implied, or not as yet clearly formulated.

These lectures on the interview present some clues regarding the not-always-easy business of getting to "know" another person, as we put it, and give some examples of the ways in which the experience of anxiety gives rise to protective patterns of behavior which invariably complicate this. In any interview a certain characteristic of speech becomes quite clear, namely that speech is used not only for the transmission of ideas but for keeping matters obscure, for the maintenance of distance from another, and for the protection by rather magical means of one's self-esteem.

One of the truly remarkable characteristics of man is his development of speech, which is so extraordinarily suited to

[1] "Affective Experience in Early Schizophrenia," *American Journal of Psychiatry* (1927) 6:467–483.

his purposes. When one observes a child, he sees a person who is interested in all that goes on about him, who is curious, who asks all manner of questions, and who uses speech as a wonderful means of getting acquainted with the world which opens out before him. Then comes the experience of anxiety in relationship with others—which is not to discount the influence of anxiety in the preverbal years—and the child discovers that certain magical qualities of speech may somehow save him from these painful decreases in his self-esteem. He learns that certain phrases such as "Excuse me," "I'm sorry," and other elaborations of words may win some semblance of approval. Thus a remarkable process occurs. At the very time when the child is expanding his knowledge of the universe and the people in it, and is beginning to acquire skill with the marvelous tool of speech—which, when joined on to his lively curiosity, will hasten that expansion—he undergoes a change which is marked by withdrawal and constriction. His curiosity is curbed, his interest in people is dulled, and he may become more concerned with the protection of his self-esteem, and with the use of language for this purpose, than with much else. This process apparently occurs to some extent in all people in our culture—and in any other of which I have any knowledge. There is almost a race between the circumstances which favor the use of language for the communication of ideas, and the circumstances favoring its use for their concealment and distortion. Should the experience of anxiety be so intense that the concealment value of language is of primary importance, there is a considerable reduction in the person's curiosity and in the possibilities of his experiencing anything like a marked realization of his potentialities. Such are those whom the psychiatrist sees as patients—and many others who never come his way. It is this remarkable intermingling of the communicative and defensive aspects of speech which characterizes every interview. This, and the background of anxiety which gives rise to it, is the central theme of these lectures.

This book stresses a certain important ingredient of successful interviewing which is frequently more adequately conveyed by gesture and tone of voice than by words. This quality or ingredient is shown by the interviewer's being keenly responsive to the needs of the interviewee, and doing nothing to lower that one's self-esteem. The skilled interviewer knows that those who come to his office have no great excess of security, and he does not become involved in heroic attempts to increase it by some magical means. That is, he does not attempt the impossible by engaging in unproductive reassuring gestures. What he does do is to demonstrate a very simple and serious respect for the other person in the interview. Now it is very impressive that such a display of honest, undecorated respect for another person brings out, in response from that other, not only reciprocal feelings of respect for the interviewer, but, most wonderfully, some feelings of increased respect for himself, the interviewee. That is exactly what one would expect to occur in a social field. When it happens in an interview, the prospects for some benefits to all concerned are excellent.

OTTO ALLEN WILL, M.D.

The Psychiatric Interview

CHAPTER
I
___

Basic Concepts in the
Psychiatric Interview

SINCE THE field of psychiatry has been defined as the study of interpersonal relations, and since it has been alleged that this is a perfectly valid area for the application of scientific method, we have come to the conclusion that the data of psychiatry arise only in participant observation. In other words, the psychiatrist cannot stand off to one side and apply his sense organs, however they may be refined by the use of apparatus, to noticing what someone else does, without becoming personally implicated in the operation. His principal instrument of observation is his self—his personality, *him* as a person. The processes and the changes in processes that make up the data which can be subjected to scientific study occur, not in the subject person nor in the observer, but in the situation which is created between the observer and his subject.

We say that the data of psychiatry arise in participant observation of social interaction, if we are inclined toward the social-psychological approach, or of interpersonal relations, if we are inclined toward the psychiatric approach, the two terms meaning, so far as I know, precisely the same thing. There are no purely objective data in psychiatry, and there are no valid subjective data, because the material becomes scientifically usable only in the shape of a complex resultant—*inference*. The vicissitudes of inference is one of the major problems in the study of psychiatry and in the development of practical psychiatric interviews.

I am not going to discuss anything like the theory of psychiatry or attempt to investigate the reasons why a good many of the things that I say seem to me to be of practical importance. In considering the subject of a serious conference with another person, I shall discuss only that which seems capable of being formulated about the steps most likely to lead to the desired end. These comments will apply whether the other person is a patient in the sense of someone seeking help for what he calls his personal idiosyncrasies, or peculiarities, or other people's strange treatment of him; whether he is someone looking for a job; or whether he has been sent by his employer to discover why he fails to make good. Any interviews calculated to meet certain criteria, which I will shortly outline, may use the same techniques as those used by the psychiatrist in attempting to discover how he can serve the professional needs of his patient. In referring to the interviewee or client, I shall sometimes speak of him as the patient, but I imply no restriction of the relevance of what I say to the medical field, believing that, for the most part, it will apply equally well to the fields of social work or personnel management, for example.

A Definition of the Psychiatric Interview

As a point of reference for comments often somewhat rambling, it may be useful to attempt a definition of what I have in mind when I speak of the psychiatric interview. As I see it, such an interview is a situation of primarily *vocal* communication in a *two-group*, more or less *voluntarily integrated*, on a progressively unfolding *expert-client* basis for the purpose of elucidating *characteristic patterns of living* of the subject person, the patient or client, which patterns he experiences as particularly troublesome or especially valuable, and in the revealing of which he expects to derive *benefit*. Of course, any person has many contacts with other people which are calculated to obtain information—if only the directions for how to get where he wants to go; but these are not properly regarded as instances of the psychiatric, or serious, highly technical inquiry.

The Vocal Nature of the Communication

The beginning of my definition of the psychiatric interview states that such an interview is a situation of primarily vocal communication—not verbal communication alone. If one assumed that everyone who came to a psychiatrist or other interviewer had to be pinned down, as one too often hears in psychiatry, or cross-examined to determine what was fact and what was fiction, then interviews would have to go on for many, many hours in order to make any sense of the other person. But if consideration is given to the nonverbal but nonetheless primarily vocal aspects of the exchange, it is actually feasible to make some sort of a crude formulation of many people in from an hour and a half to, let us say, six hours of serious discourse (I might add, not six consecutive hours, though I've even done that). Much attention may profitably be paid to the telltale aspects of intonation, rate of speech, difficulty in enunciation, and so on—factors which are conspicuous to any student of vocal communication. It is by alertness to the importance of these things as signs or indicators of meaning, rather than by preoccupation only with the words spoken, that the psychiatric interview becomes practical in a reasonable section of one's lifetime.

The experience that gives me a peculiar, if not an important, slant on this whole matter is that I was initially intensely interested in schizophrenic patients. Schizophrenics are very shy people, low in self-esteem and subject to the suspicion that they are not particularly appreciated or respected by strangers. Like many other people, they are rather sensitive to scrutiny, to inspection, and to being "looked in the eye." Perhaps in all too many cases they are full of ancient traditional hokum from the culture about the eyes being the windows of the soul, and things being seen in them that might not otherwise be revealed —which seems to be one of the most misguided ideas I've ever known. In brief, schizophrenics are embarrassed by being stared at.

As I wished to learn as much as I could about schizophrenics (and with good fortune, perhaps about other humans as well), I very early in my psychiatric research work abandoned the idea of watching people while they talked with me. For years, seven and a half at least, I sat at an angle of ninety degrees from the people whom I interviewed, and usually gazed at something quite definitely in front of me—very clearly not at them. Since the field of vision is so great that one can observe motor movement in another person over an extraordinarily wide range, I think I missed few of my patients' starts, sudden changes of posture, and one thing and another, but certainly I could not see the fine movements of their faces.[1]

In order to become somewhat at ease about what was going on, I necessarily developed further an already considerable auditory acuity so that I could hear the kind of things which, perhaps, most people are inclined to deceive themselves into thinking that they can only see. I do believe that the majority of clues to what people actually mean reach us via the ears. Tonal variations in the voice—and by "tonal variations" I mean, very broadly and generically, changes in all the complex group of things that make up speech—are frequently wonderfully dependable clues to shifts in the communicative situation. For example, if somebody is attempting to describe his work as a journeyman electrician, things may go on quite well until he is on the verge of saying something about the job which pertains to a field in which he has been guilty of gross disloyalty to his union, at which time his voice will sound altered. He may still give the facts about what a journeyman electrician should be and do, but he will sound different in the telling.

[1] A visual study to determine what there is about other people's faces that gives away falsehoods and so on immediately demonstrates the gross absurdity of thinking that their eyes provide us with any clues. Even in the lower part of the face, which is distinctly more expressive and closely related to the mental state of the person concerned, the tensions are not by any means so labile that they keep up with the changing mixture of truth, best appearances, untruth, and frank falsehood that make up a great deal of communication.

In the psychiatric interview a great part of the experience which one slowly gains manifests itself in a show of mild interest in the point at which there is a tonal difference. Thus the interviewer would perhaps say, "Oh, yes, and the payment of exactly 2½ per cent of one's income to this fund for the sick and wounded is almost never neglected by good union members, I gather"; to which the other might reply, again sounding quite different from the way he had earlier, "Exactly! It's a very important part of membership." And then, if the interviewer feels sure of the situation, he might say, "And one, of course, which you have never violated." Whereupon the other person sounds very different indeed, perhaps quite indignant, and says, "Of course not!" If the interviewer is extremely sure of the way things are going, he might even say, "Well, of course you understand I have no suspicion about you, but your voice sounded odd when you mentioned it, and I couldn't help but wonder if it was preying on your mind." At this the other person may sound still more different, and say, "Well, as a matter of fact, early in my journeymanship I actually did pocket a little of the percentage, and it has been on my conscience ever since."

Thus the psychiatric interview is primarily a matter of vocal communication, and it would be a quite serious error to presume that the communication is primarily verbal. The sound-accompaniments suggest what is to be made of the verbal propositions stated. Of course, a great many of these verbal propositions may be taken as simply matters of routine data, subject to the ordinary probabilities and to such further inquiries as will make clear what the person means.

I do not believe that I have had an interview with anybody in twenty-five years in which the person to whom I was talking was not annoyed during the early part of the interview by my asking stupid questions—I am certain that I usually correctly read the patient's mind in this respect. A patient tells me the obvious and I wonder what he means, and ask further questions. But after the first half-hour or so, he begins to see that there is a reasonable uncertainty as to what he meant, and that statements which seem obvious to him may be remarkably uncommunicative to the other person. They may be far worse than uncommunicative, for they may permit the inexperienced interviewer to assume that he knows something that is not the case. Only belatedly does he discover that he has been galloping off on a little path of private fantasy which clearly could not be what the patient was talking about, because now the patient is talking about something so obviously irrelevant to it. Thus part of the skill in interviewing comes from a sort of quiet observation all along: "Does this sentence, this statement, have an unquestionable meaning? Is there any certainty as to what this person means?"

For example, during an interview one may learn that a person is married, and if one is feeling very mildly satirical, one can say, "And doubtless happily?" If the answer is "Yes," that "Yes" can have anything in the way of implication from a dirge to a paean of supreme joy. It may indicate that the "Yes" means "No," or anything in between. The logical question, I suppose, after learning how happily the person is married, might be, "Was it your first love?" The answer may be "Yes," at which one may say, "Is that so? That's most unusual." Now, nobody cares whether it's most unusual or not. In fact, it is *fairly* unusual, but it isn't *most* unusual. The "most unusual" makes it an issue, with the result that the informant feels that it requires a little explanation; he is not quite sure whether or not it is something to be proud of. And at this point the interviewer may begin to hear a little about the interviewee's history of interpersonal intimacy with the other sex. Frequently, for example, in cases of marriage to the first love, there is a very open question of whether love has ever entered the patient's life, and one discovers that the marriage is nothing very delightful.

The Two-Group

To return to my definition of the interview, the next point is that this communication is in a two-group, and in that suggestion there certainly is a faint measure of irony. While it is practically impossible to explore most of the significant areas of personality with a third person present. it is also true that even though only two people are actually in the room, the number of more or less imaginary people that get themselves involved in this two-group is sometimes really hair-raising. In fact, two or three times in the course of an hour, or more, whole new sets of these imaginary others may also be present in the field. Of that, more later when I discuss what I call parataxic distortion.

Voluntary Integration of the Participants

The next point I would like to make concerns the patient's more or less voluntary entrance into this therapeutic situation on an expert-client basis. Psychiatrists are accustomed to dealing with people of all degrees of willingness, all the way from those who are extremely unwilling to see them but are required to do so by process of law, to those who are seriously interested in getting the benefits of modern psychiatry. I think that these startling extremes only accentuate the fact that probably most people go into any interview with quite mixed motivations; they wish that they could talk things over frankly with somebody, but they also carry with them, practically from childhood, ingrained determinations which block free discussion. As a result, people often expect that the psychiatrist will be either a great genius or a perfect ass.

Now, the other side of the picture: There are some more or less voluntary elements in the psychiatrist's attitude. He may vary from enthusiasm for what he is about to discover, to a bored indifference about the patient—and these attitudes unhappily may be determined very early in the interview. The attitudes of the interviewee are data. But any striking emotion on the part of the interviewer is an unhappy artifact which amounts to a psychiatric problem. For example, any intense curiosity about the details of another person's life, particularly his sexual life or drinking habits, or something like that, is a very unfortunate ingredient in a psychiatric interview. On the other hand, a more or less disdainful indifference to what the patient may have to offer amounts to a quite serious evidence of morbidity on the part of an interviewer.

As I shall presently suggest, there is no fun in psychiatry. If you try to get fun out of it, you pay a considerable price for your unjustifiable optimism. If you do not feel equal to the headaches that psychiatry induces, you are in the wrong business. It is work—work the like of which I do not know. True, it ordinarily does not require vast physical exertion, but it does require a high degree of alertness to a sometimes very rapidly shifting field of signs which are remarkably complex in themselves and in their relations. And the necessity for promptness of response to what happens proves in the course of a long day to be very tiring indeed. It is curious, but there are data that suggest that the more complicated the field to which one must attend, the more rapidly fatigue sets in. For example, in dealing with a serious problem in a very competent person, the psychiatrist will find that grasping the nuances of what is reserved, and what is distorted, and what is unknown by the communicant but very relevant to the work at hand, is not easy. So an enthusiasm about psychiatry is preposterous—it shows one just hasn't grown up; but at the same time, for the psychiatrist to be indifferent toward his work is fatal. The more dependable attitude of the psychiatrist in a psychiatric interview is probably simply to have a very serious realization that he is earning his living, and that he must work for it.

Whether the patient thinks at the beginning that he is very eager to see the psychiatrist or the interviewer, or whether he thinks he is bitterly opposed to it all, is less important. This does make some slight difference at the start, because one tries to accommodate, insofar as one readily can, to the mood of the patient. In other words, if a person comes to you quite angrily, it is not particularly helpful to beam on him and say, "Why, my dear fellow, you seem upset. Do tell me what's troubling you!" That is probably too reminiscent of the worst of his past experience with maiden aunts and so on. When people approach you angrily, you take them very seriously, and, if you're like me, with the faint suggestion that you can be angry too, and that you would like to know what the shooting is about.

Thus the initial attitude—be it willingness or unwillingness, hesitancy or reservation—of the client determines somewhat the attitude, and perhaps the pattern, of the interviewer's initial inquiries. But the client's attitude is not in itself to be taken very seriously; many very resistant people prove to be remarkably communicative as soon as they discover that the interrogator makes some sense and that he is not simply distributing praise, blame, and so on.

The Expert-Client Relationship

The expert-client relationship, which I have mentioned, implies a good deal. As defined in this culture, the expert is one who derives his income and status, one or both, from the use of unusually exact or adequate information about his particular field, in the service of others. This "use in the service of" is fixed in our industrial-commercial social order. The expert does not trade in the implements or impedimenta of his field; he is not a 'merchant,' a 'collector,' a 'connoisseur,' or a 'fancier,' for these use their skill primarily in their own interest.

The psychiatric expert is expected to have an unusual grasp on the field of interpersonal relations, and, since this problem-area is peculiarly the field of participant observation, the psychiatrist is expected to manifest extraordinary skill in the relationship with his subject-person or patient. Insofar as all those who come to him must be by definition relatively insecure, the psychiatrist is peculiarly estopped from seeking personal satisfactions or prestige at their expense. He seeks only the data needed to benefit the patient, and expects to be paid for this service.

By and large, any expert who traffics in the commodities about which he is supposed to be an expert runs the risk of being called a fancier, or a connoisseur, or a sharper, or something of that kind. This is because people are at a peculiar disadvantage in dealing with the expert who has an extraordinary grasp on a field; and if he traffics in the commodities concerned, as well as in the skill, people are afraid and suspicious of him. By cultural definition, they expect him to be a purveyor of exact information and skill, and to have no connection with the commercial-industrial world other than to be paid for such services. This is poignantly the case with psychiatrists, who work in a field the complexity of which is so intimidating that very few of them maintain for long the conceit that they are great experts at psychiatry. It is very striking to consider the cultural definition of the expert as it applies to the psychiatrist: he is an *expert* having *expert* knowledge of interpersonal relations, personality problems, and so on; he has no traffic in the satisfactions which may come from interpersonal relations, and he does not pursue prestige or standing in the eyes of his clients, or at the expense of his clients. In accordance with this definition, the psychiatrist is quite obviously uninterested in what the patient might have to offer, temporarily or permanently, as a companion, and quite resistant to any support by the patient for his prestige, importance, and so on.

It is only if the psychiatrist is very clearly aware of this taboo, as it were, on trafficking in the ordinary commodities of interpersonal relations, that many suspicious people discover that they can deal with him and can actually communicate to him their problems with other people. Thus the psychiatrist must be keenly aware of this particular aspect of the expert's role—that he deals primarily in information, in correct, unusually adequate information, and that he is estopped by the cultural attitude from using his expert knowledge to get himself personal satisfaction, or to obviously enhance his prestige or reputation at the expense of the patient. Only if he is keenly aware of this can the expert-client relationship in this field be consolidated rapidly and with reasonable ease.

The Patient's Characteristic Patterns of Living

To return again to my definition of the psychiatric interview, I said that it is for the purpose of elucidating characteristic patterns of living. Personality very strikingly demonstrates in every instance, in every situation, the perduring effects of the past; and the effects of a particular past event are not only perhaps fortunate or unfortunate, but also extensively intertwined with the effects of a great many other past events. Thus there is no such thing as learning what *ails* a person's living, in the sense that you will come to know anything definite, without getting a pretty good idea of who it is that's doing the living, and with whom. In other words, in every case, whether you know it or not, if you are to correctly understand your patient's problems, you must understand him in the major characteristics of his dealing with people. Now, this relationship of difficulty in living to all the rest of the important characteristics of a personality is a thing which I must stress, because we are such capable creatures, we humans, that we do not always know anywhere near what we have experienced. Psychiatrists know a great deal about their patients that they don't know they know. For example, caught off guard by the offhand question of a friendly colleague— "Yes, but damn his difficulties in living! What sort of *person* is this patient of yours?"—the psychiatrist may rattle off a description that would do him honor if he only knew it.

And do you think that this is restricted to psychiatrists? What you know about the people whom you know at all well is truly amazing, even though you have never formulated it. It may never have been very important for you to formulate it; it hasn't been worth anything to you, you might say. All that it's worth, of course, is that it makes for better understanding; but, if your interest lies in what the person does and not in understanding him, you probably don't know how much you know about him.

In the psychiatric interview, it is a very good idea to know as much as possible about the patient. It is very much easier to do therapy if the patient has caught on to the fact that you are interested in understanding something of what he thinks ails him, and also what sort of person his more admiring friends regard him to be, and so on. Thus the purpose of the interview is to elucidate the characteristic patterns of living, some of which make trouble for the patient.

Many people who consult psychiatrists regard themselves as the victims of disease, or hereditary defect, or God knows what in the way of some sort of evil, fateful entity that is tied to them or built into them. They don't think of their troubles, as they call them, as important, but not especially distinguished, parts of their general performance of living in a civilized world with other people. Many problems are so thoroughly removed from any connection with other people—when they are reported by the patient—that the young psychiatrist would, I think, feel rather timid about suggesting to the patient that perhaps he did not experience these problems in his relations with everybody, but only with some particular people; and I think that even the very experienced psychiatrist would scarcely wish to expose the patient to such unnecessary stress. But one can always ask *when* the trouble occurs—in what setting it is most likely to be seen. Remarkably often one of these patients who has an "organic" or "hereditary" neurosis that has nothing to do with other people can produce instances of his neurosis in which five or six different people have been involved—and for the life of him can't think of any other settings in which it has been demonstrated. It is only when he has come to this point that the psychiatrist can say, "In other words, you don't have this difficulty, so far as you know, with your wife and her maiden sister, and so on and so forth?" The patient stops, and thinks, and quite honestly says, "No, I don't believe I ever do." Only then is he on the verge of realizing that perhaps the other fellow *does* have something to do with the difficulty; only after being led around to making that discovery from his own data can he begin to realize that it is the interpersonal context that calls out many troubles.

I am not attempting to say here that there is nothing that makes living difficult except other people and one's inadequate preparation for dealing with them. There are a vast number of things, such as blindness in one or both eyes, and harelip, and poor education, which make difficulties in living. But the psychiatric interview is primarily designed to discover *obscure* difficulties in living which the patient does not clearly understand: in other words, that which for cultural reasons—reasons of his particular education for life—he is foggy about, chronically misleads himself about, or misleads others about. Such difficulties stand out more clearly and more meaningfully as one grasps what sort of a person he is, and what that person does, and why.

To sum up, a patient's patterns of difficulty arise in his past experience and variously interpenetrate all aspects of his current interpersonal relationships. Without data reflecting many important aspects of the patient's personality, the patient's statement of symptoms and the psychiatrist's observation of signs of difficulty are unintelligible.

The Patient's Expectation of Benefit

This brings me to the final portion of my definition—that the patient has at least some expectation of improvement or other personal gain from the interview. This statement may not sound particularly impressive; yet I have participated in long interviews that have been very unpleasant to the patient but which have come to some end useful to him and satisfactory to me only because he caught on to the fact that there was something in it for him. The *quid pro quo* which keeps people going in this necessarily disturbing business of trying to be foursquare and straightforward about one's most lamentable failures and one's most chagrining mistakes is that one is learning something that promises to be useful. Insofar as the patient's participation in the interview situation inspires in the patient a conviction that the psychiatrist is learning not only *how* the patient has trouble, but *who* the patient is and *with whom* he has trouble, the implied expectation of benefit is in process of realization.

I wish to put a good deal of emphasis on this, because there are interview situations in which there is no attention paid whatever to what the interrogee—the victim, one might say—gets out of it. Instead, it is a wholly one-sided interrogation. Questions are asked and the answers are received by a person who pays no attention at all to the anxiety or the feeling of insecurity of the informant, and who gives no clue to the meaning of the information elicited. These one-sided interrogations are all right for certain very limited and crudely defined purposes. For example, if you want to accumulate in fifteen minutes some clues as to whether or not a person will probably survive two years in the Army under any circumstances that are apt to transpire in two years in the Army, then you can use this type of interrogation. But, out of a large number of people interviewed in this way, the percentage of error in your judgment will be high. How high this percentage is, nobody has yet very adequately determined, for even the people who set out to use one-sided interrogation undoubtedly interpret a good deal that goes on besides the answering itself.

One can, in a rather brief interview, reach certain limited objectives. For example, an interviewer can determine that a person should not be given a job as a telephone operator by discovering that he has no capacity for righting himself after a misunderstanding, or that he is unnerved by someone's being unpleasant to him. But for purposes anything like those of the psychiatric interview, in which one is actually attempting to assess a person's assets and liabilities in terms of his future living, some time is required, and a simple question-answer technique will not work.

The interviewer must be sure that the other person is getting something out of it, that his expectation of improving himself (as he may put it), of getting a better job, or of attaining whatever has motivated him in undergoing the interview, gets encouragement. As long as this personal objective receives support, the communicative situation improves, and the interviewer comes finally to have data on which he can make a formulation of some value to himself as an expert, and to the other person concerned.

To sum up, the psychiatric interview, as considered here, is primarily a two-group in which there is an expert-client relationship, the expert being defined by the culture. Insofar as there is such an expert-client relationship, the interviewee expects the person who sits behind the desk to show a really

expert grasp on the intricacies of interpersonal relations; he
expects the interviewer to show skill in conducting the interview. The greater this skill, other things being equal, the more
easily will the purpose of the interview be achieved. The interviewer must discover who the client is—that is, he must review
what course of events the client has come through to be who
he is, what he has in the way of background and experience.
And, on the basis of who the person is, the interviewer must
learn what this person conceives of in his living as problematic,
and what he feels to be difficult. This is true whether one is
interviewing with the primary idea of finding the person a
doctor, of curing him of a so-called mental disorder, of getting
him a job, of placing him in a factory, of separating him from
some type of service, or of deciding whether he can be trusted
in a certain position. In finding out in what areas the interviewee
has his trouble in functioning, the interviewer would do well
to remember that no matter how vastly superior a person may
be, there is enough in the culture to justify his having some
trouble. I have rarely experienced the embarrassment, or the
privilege, of being consulted by a person who had no troubles,
and I may say that when this did appear to be the case, it rapidly
proved to be an artifact. Thus we may assume that everybody
has some trouble in living; I think it is ordained by our social
order itself that none of us can find and maintain a way of life
with perfect contentment, proper self-respect, and so on.

The interviewer's learning wherein his client encounters
headaches in dealing with his fellow man and achieving the
purposes of his life, which is of the essence of the psychiatric
interview, implies that the other fellow must get something in
exchange for what he gives. The *quid pro quo* which leads to
the best psychiatric interview—as well as the best interview
for employment or for other purposes—is that the person being
interviewed realizes, quite early, that he is going to learn something useful about the way he lives. In such circumstances, he
may very well become communicative; otherwise, he will show
as much caution as his intellect and background permit, giving
no information that he conceives might in any way do him

harm. To repeat, that the person will leave with some measure of increased clarity about himself and his living with other people is an essential goal of the psychiatric interview.

The Psychiatrist as a Participant Observer

As I said at the beginning, psychiatry is peculiarly the field of participant observation. The fact is that we cannot make any sense of, for example, the motor movements of another person except on the basis of behavior that is meaningful to us—that is, on the basis of what we have experienced, done ourselves, or seen done under circumstances in which its purpose, its motivation, or at least the intentions behind it were communicated to us. Without this past background, the observer cannot deduce, by sheer intellectual operations, the meaning of the staggering array of human acts. As an example of this, almost all the things pertaining to communication form such highly conventionalized patterns and are so fixed within the culture that if my pronunciation of a word deviates from yours, you may wonder what in the world I am talking about. Things having to do with your own past experience and with proscriptions of the culture and so on that were common in your home; activities which are attached to you as the person concerned in their doing, and activities to which you respond as if you were the person primarily, directly, and simply concerned in them—all these are the data of psychiatry. Therefore, the psychiatrist has an inescapable, inextricable involvement in all that goes on in the interview; and to the extent that he is unconscious or unwitting of his participation in the interview, to that extent he does not know what is happening. This is another argument in favor of the position that the psychiatrist has a hard enough job to do without any pursuit of his own pleasure or prestige. He can legitimately expect only the satisfaction of feeling that he did what he was paid for—that will be enough, and probably more than he can do well.

The psychiatrist should never lose track of the fact that all the processes of the patient are more or less exactly addressed at him, and that all that he offers—his experience—is more or less accurately aimed at the patient, with a resulting wonderful interplay. For example, one realizes that statements are not things that can be rigidly fixed as to meaning by Webster's or the Oxford Dictionary, but that they are only approximations, sometimes remote approximations, of what is meant. But that is just the beginning of the complexities of the participant character of the psychiatric interview—for that matter, of all attempts at communication between people, of which the psychiatric interview is an especially characterized example.

That does not mean, as some of our experts in semantics might lead us to suppose, that before a psychiatrist starts talking with his patient he should give him a list of words that are not to be used. It simply means, as I said earlier, that the psychiatrist listens to all statements with a certain critical interest, asking, "Could that mean anything except what first occurs to me?" He questions (at least to himself) much of what he hears, not on the assumption that the patient is a liar, or doesn't know how to express himself, or anything like that, but always with the simple query in mind, "Now, could this mean something that would not immediately occur to me? Do I know what he means by that?" Every now and then this leads to the interviewer's asking questions aloud, but it certainly does not imply the vocal questioning of every statement. So if the patient says, "The milkman dropped a can of milk last night and it woke me up," I am usually willing to presume that it is simply so.

On the other hand, a patient may say, "Well, he's my dearest friend! He hasn't a hostile impulse toward me!" I then assume that this is to explain in some curious fashion that this other person has done him an extreme disservice, such as running away with his wife—or perhaps it was a great service; I have yet to discover, from the interview, which it was. And I say, "Is that so? It sounds amazing." Now when I say a thing sounds amazing, the patient feels very much on the spot; he feels that he must prove something, and he tells me more about how wonderful his friend's motivation is. Having heard still more, I am able to say, "Well, is it possible that you can think of nothing he ever did that was at least unfortunate in its effect?" At this the poor fellow will no doubt remember the elopement of his wife. And thus we gradually come to discover why it is necessary for him to consider this other person to be such a perfect friend—quite often a very illuminating field to explore. God knows, it may be the nearest approach to a good friend this man has ever had, and he feels exceedingly the need of a friend.

The more conventional a person's statements are, of course, the more doubtful it is that you have any idea of what he really means. For example, there are people who have been trained to cultivate virtue (and the cultural motives that provided this training were horrible) to such an extent that they are truly almost incapable of saying any evil of anybody.

The psychiatrist, the interviewer, plays a very active role in introducing interrogations, not to show that he is smart or that he is skeptical, but literally to make sure that he knows what he is being told. Few things do the patient more good in the way of getting toward his more or less clearly formulated desire to benefit from the investigation than this very care on the part of the interviewer to discover exactly what is meant. Almost every time one asks, "Well, do you mean so and so?" the patient is a little clearer on what he does mean. And what a relief it is to him to discover that his true meaning is anything but what he at first says, and that he is at long last uncovering some conventional self-deception that he has been pulling on himself for years.

Let me illustrate this last by telling you of a young man who had been clearly sinking into a schizophrenic illness for several months and who was referred to me by a colleague. Among the amazing things I extracted from this poor citizen was that, to his amazement and chagrin, he spent a good deal of his time in the kitchen with his mother making dirty cracks at her, saying either obscure or actually bitter and critical things to her. He thought he must be crazy, because he was the only child and his mother, so he said, was perfect. As a matter of fact, he had two perfect parents. They had done everything short of carrying him around on a pillow. And now he had broken down just because he was engaged in a couple of full-time courses at one of our best universities. In other words, he was a bright boy, and had very healthy ambitions which represented the realization of the very fine training that he had been given by these excellent parents. I undertook to discover what was so surprising to him about this business of his hostile remarks to his mother, and he made it quite clear that the surprising thing was that she had never done him any harm, and had actually enfolded him in every kind of good. To all this I thought, "Oh yeah? It doesn't sound so to me. It doesn't make sense. Maybe you have overlooked something."

By that time I was actually able to say something like this: "I have a vague feeling that some people might doubt the utility to you of the care with which your parents, and particularly your mother, saw to it that you didn't learn how to dance, or play games, or otherwise engage in the frivolous social life of people of your age." And I was delighted to see the schizophrenic young man give me a sharp look. Although he was seated where I didn't have to look directly at him, I could see that. And I said, "Or was that an unmitigated blessing?" There was a long pause, and then he opined that when he was young he might have been sore about it.

I guessed that that wasn't the whole story—that he was still sore about it, and with very good reason. Then I inquired if he had felt any disadvantage in college from the lack of these social skills with which his colleagues whiled away their evenings, and so on. He recalled that he had often noticed his defects in that field, and that he regretted them. With this improvement in intelligence, we were able to glean more of what the mother had actually done and said to discourage his impulse to develop social techniques. At the end of an hour and a half devoted more or less entirely to this subject, I was able to say, "Well, now, is it really so curious that you're being unpleasant to your mother?" And he thought that perhaps it wasn't.

A couple of days later the family telephoned to say that he was greatly benefited by his interview with me. As a matter of fact, he unquestionably was. But the benefit—and this is perhaps part of why I tell the story—arose from the discovery that a performance of his, which was deeply distressing to him because it seemed irrational and entirely unjust, became reasonably justified by a change in his awareness of his past and of his relationship with the present victim of his behavior. Thus the feeling was erased that he was crazy, that only a madman would be doing this—and, believe me, it is no help to anybody's peace of mind to feel that he is mad. His peace of mind was enhanced to the extent that it was no longer necessary for him to feel chagrin, contempt for himself, and all sorts of dim religious impiety; but on the other hand he could feel, as I attempted to suggest in our initial interview, that there wasn't anything different in his behavior from practically anybody else's except the accents in the patterns of its manifestation. As he was able to comprehend that the repulsive, queer, strange, mystifying, chagrining, horrifying aspects of his experience reflected defects in his memory and understanding concerning its origins, the necessity to manifest the behavior appeared to diminish, which actually meant that competing processes were free to appear, and that the partitioning of his life was to some degree broken down. The outwardly meaningless, psychotic attacks on his mother did not give him the satisfaction that came from asking her more directly why in the devil she had never let him learn to play bridge. With the substitution of the possibility of a more direct approach, the psychotic material disappeared and he was better.

Thus whenever the psychiatrist's attempt to discover what the patient is talking about leads the patient to be somewhat more clear on what he is thinking about or attempting to communicate or conceal, his grasp on life is to some extent enhanced. And no one has grave difficulties in living if he has a very good grasp on what is happening to him.

Everything in that sentence depends on what I mean by "grave," and let me say that here I am referring to those difficulties unquestionably requiring the intervention of an expert. It is my opinion that man is rather staggeringly endowed with adaptive capacities, and I am quite certain that when a person is clear on the situation in which he finds himself, he does one of three things: he decides it is too much for him and leaves it, he handles it satisfactorily, or he calls in adequate help to handle it. And that's all there is to it.

When people find themselves recurrently in obscure situations which they feel they should understand and actually don't, and in which they feel that their prestige requires them to take adequate action (a somewhat hypothetical entity, since they do not know what the situation is), they are clearly in need of psychiatric assistance. That assistance is by way of the participant observation of the psychiatrist and the patient, in which the psychiatrist attempts to discover what is happening to the patient. A great many questions may be asked and answered in the psychiatric interview before the patient sees much of what the psychiatrist is exploring; but, in the process, the patient will have experienced many beginning clarifications of matters which will subsequently take on considerable personal significance.

As an example of such an obscure situation which seemed to demand action, I would like to mention a patient whom I saw for a brief interview a number of years ago in New York. She was a young lady of forty-three or so who presented, as her trouble in life, the fact that at night her breasts were frightfully tampered with by her sister who lived in Oklahoma. Now, such a statement is a reasonable sign of something being a little the matter with the mind. It also developed that the pastor of one of the more important New York churches gave the only help that she had ever been able to obtain in this cursed nuisance perpetrated by her sister. Since I always appreciate any help that anybody can get, particularly from somebody besides me, I was pleased to learn this and wondered why she had sought me out.

At this I learned that there were other difficulties. She was coming to suspect that a woman who worked in her office had been employed by her sister to spy on her—this nice psychotic lady, like many others, was earning a living. I said, "Aha! Now we are getting somewhere! Tell me all about that." Whereupon she bridled, realizing that it was risky to admit

psychotic content to a psychiatrist. It developed that she had
been controlling increasing rage against this woman in her
office for weeks, and that she had been consulting her pastor
with increasing frequency about the problem. I didn't ask what
he did. But I did happen to look at the clock at that point and
discovered that I had been keeping another patient waiting
twenty minutes. So I said to the young lady, "Well, look here.
I don't believe it would be practicable for me to attempt to
substitute for the friendly adviser who is considerable comfort
and support to you. But I do want to say one thing, which I
have to say both as a psychiatrist and as a member of society: If
you feel impelled to do something physical to square yourself
with this persecutor in your office, then, madam, before you do
it, go to the psychopathic pavilion at Bellevue and apply for
voluntary admission for two or three days. In the end that will
be much better." And she said, "Oh, you're like all the other
psychiatrists!" With which the interview was over. I am quite
certain that she derived considerable benefit from the finish of
that interview.

The Concept of Parataxic Distortion

Now let us notice a feature of all interpersonal relations
which is especially striking in the intimate type of inquiry
which the psychiatric interview can be, and which is, in fact,
strangely illustrated in the case I have just mentioned. This is
the parataxic, as I call it, concomitant in life. By this I mean
that not only are there quite tangible people involved (in this
case the patient's sister living in Oklahoma and a fellow employee in the patient's office), but also somewhat fantastic
constructs of those people are involved, such as the sister tin-
kering with the patient's breasts in her Manhattan room at
night, and the fellow employee acting as an emissary or agent
of her sister. These psychotic elaborations of imaginary people
and imaginary personal performances are spectacular and seem
very strange. But the fact is that in a great many relationships
of the most commonplace kind—with neighbors, enemies, acquaintances, and even such statistically determined people as

the collector and the mailman—variants of such distortions often exist. The characteristics of a person that would be agreed to by a large number of competent observers may not appear to you to be the characteristics of the person toward whom you are making adjustive or maladjustive movements. The *real* characteristics of the other fellow at that time may be of negligible importance to the interpersonal situation. This we call *parataxic distortion*.

Parataxic distortion as a term may sound quite unusual; actually the phenomena it describes are anything but unusual. The great complexity of the psychiatric interview is brought about by the interviewee's substituting for the psychiatrist a person or persons strikingly different in most significant respects from the psychiatrist. The interviewee addresses his behavior toward this fictitious person who is temporarily in the ascendancy over the reality of the psychiatrist, and he interprets the psychiatrist's remarks and behavior on the basis of this same fictitious person. There are often clues to the occurrence of these phenomena. Such phenomena are the basis for the really astonishing misunderstandings and misconceptions which characterize all human relations, and certain special precautions must be taken against them in the psychiatric interview after it is well under way. Parataxic distortion is also one way that the personality displays before another some of its gravest problems. In other words, parataxic distortion may actually be an obscure attempt to communicate something that really needs to be grasped by the therapist, and perhaps finally to be grasped by the patient. Needless to say, if such distortions go unnoted, if they are not expected, if the possibility of their existence is ignored, some of the most important things about the psychiatric interview may go by default.

CHAPTER
II

The Structuring of the
Interview Situation

The Cultural Role of the
Psychiatrist as an Expert

I HAVE ALREADY stressed the cultural definition of an expert. I now want to discuss further the peculiar aspects of that definition as it applies to the psychiatrist, or to anyone who functions in the general field of the psychiatrist—that is, to a serious student of, shall I say, practical aspects of human personality and living.

I think that what society teaches one to expect is important. The person who comes to the interview expecting a certain pattern of events which does not materialize will probably not return; he will not say nice things about the interviewer if the latter, feeling that the things expected by his client are irrelevant or immaterial, ignores these expectations and presents the client with something much "better." In other words, what a client is taught to expect is the thing that he should get—or, at least, any variation should very clearly depart from it in a rather carefully arranged way. To illustrate, a person comes to you expecting the satisfaction, let us say, of a thirst for contentment. You may feel, in contrast, that it would be a great thing for him to learn how to make a living. But, before you expect success in offering him help in making a living, please pay attention to the fact that he is there to gain contentment, and that you will have to take what he expects into consideration if you wish to wean him from his interest in contentment and induce him to follow you in developing an interest in making a living. The social or cultural definition is very important indeed in the earlier stages of an interpersonal relation; in fact, it is finally important if one of the people concerned overlooks it, since this means that the relationship will not be developed in any meaningful sense. Something will happen, but the person who has overlooked the cultural definition of the situation will not know what has happened, and the course of events thereafter will not particularly suit him. The psychiatric expert, or anyone who sees a stranger on the assumption that he will find out about him and possibly be useful to him, may well pay considerable attention to what is traditionally, in informed society, accepted as the function of one in his particular expert role.

Let me mention now some of the ways in which the psychiatrist, in his work, illustrates this social definition. The psychiatric expert is expected to have an unusual grasp on the field of interpersonal relations, one which is very extensive, or very wonderfully detailed, or both. He is supposed to be at least somewhat familiar with practically everything that people do one with another, and to know more than his client does about the interpersonal relations in any field of interest that may be discussed. He is supposed to have such an unusual grasp on the technique of participant observation that when he talks with another person, he learns more than could be expected of any reasonably intelligent ordinary mortal. He catches on to more; he is more informed about what goes on in his relations with others than are even really talented, but not expertly trained, people. And he is expected to show his expertness in the management of his relation with the patient—an expectation in which many patients are woefully disappointed now and then. In other words, since the psychiatrist is an expert in interpersonal relations, it is not at all strange that the patient comes to the physician expecting him to handle things so that the patient's purpose will be served: namely, that his assets and liabilities in living will be correctly appraised, and that his difficulties will be tracked down to meaningful and remediable elements in his past—or that he will be advised, for instance, to divorce his wife in case she is really his trouble instead of his past. The psychiatric expert is presumed, from the cultural definition of an expert, and from the general rumors and beliefs about psychiatry, to be quite able to handle a psychiatric interview.

Now this statement implies that the demonstration of expertness in the psychiatric interview takes place, as Adolf Meyer once said, in the "here and now" of that interview. It does not take place somewhere else—for example, in the office of the physician who says, "You ought to see a psychiatrist, and I think so-and-so is a marvelous psychiatrist." That is all right; it may get the patient into the subway, or over the bus system, on his way to the psychiatrist's office, but it does nothing to establish the expert-client relationship which is the underlying factor in the possibilities of success of the psychiatric interview. The psychiatrist must demonstrate to the patient, in terms of the rumors and beliefs prevalent in the particular stratum of society from which the patient comes, that the psychiatrist is at least something of the person he is expected to be.

The psychiatrist demonstrates that he fulfills the expected role—insofar as these expectations make any sense and have any significance at all—if the patient experiences, in the course of the interview, something that impresses him as a really expert capacity for handling him, the patient. If you will pause to consider the people whom you look upon as "understanding"—that is, able to handle you expertly—you will notice that they demonstrate a very considerable respect for you. Meeting such a person can be a really significant event; it is almost a privilege to have him around. This respect for you, which is so impressive when experienced, not only takes the general form of endorsing your worth as a companion in the same room, but is also shown by a certain warning of any severe jolts that you might receive in the discussion, and by a certain tendency to come to your rescue at those junctures at which you would feel better if you had some information that you don't happen to have, and so on and so forth. In other words, you are well managed, first, when you are treated as worth the trouble, and second, when the other person is keenly aware of, and sensitive to, disturbances in your feeling of personal worth, in your security, while in his presence.

Thus when a certain question is going to touch on a topic or field regarding which the patient feels insecure or anxious, the psychiatrist makes a little preliminary movement which indicates that he is quite aware of the unpleasantness that will attend this question, but also that it is obviously necessary that he should know the information; in other words, he gives the patient a little warning to brace himself. Now and then he may recognize that the patient is anxious about something which to the psychiatrist seems to be among the most natural things on earth; at that point he may say, "Well, do you feel that that's unusual?" The patient may say, "Well, yes, I'm afraid I do"; and the psychiatrist replies, "Dear me! Why, I never heard anybody talk honestly who didn't mention that." Thus respect for the other person, and awareness of the other person's feeling of security, is the first element of the expertness in interpersonal relations which any client will look for in an interviewer who is engaged in a psychiatric or quasi-psychiatric task. And if the client does not find it, no amount of propaganda by the family physician is going to make it look to him like a good situation, or make the results of the interview very deeply illuminating.

RELEVANT AND IRRELEVANT DATA

Both the culture and the social order—what is taught from the cradle onward—may support the psychiatrist in saying that as an expert he is "entitled to" or has a "right to" certain relevant and significant data about the person who consults him. In other words, such data are necessary on the basic assumption that the psychiatrist must understand who the client is and how things happened in his life. Anyone's being "entitled to" or having a "right to" anything is, of course, a very obscure reference to something very complicated. But so prevalent is this notion that there are inherent and indwelling rights connected with you, your family, your job, and so on, ad infinitum, that the client usually accepts it. The social order is such that no sooner do you as a psychiatrist indicate this assumption than the overwhelming movement in the client's personality is toward the conclusion: "Why, of course, the doctor is entitled to it. He must have it to make any sense of this problem of mine." And thus the psychiatrist engages in no arguments concerning the "right" or "wrong" of his being given data, or in debates relating to the "propriety" of his hearing this or that, or the "necessity" for the patient to reveal thus and so. He simply assumes that data must be given in order to make any sense at all of the always much too obscure processes of living; he avoids extended discussions with his patient about the origins of or the reasons for the assumption, presenting it as a sort of dogma, to be accepted of necessity if the work is to go forward and make any sense at all. Of course, if the patient does not accept this assumption, and wants to know what in the world I'm talking about, I tell him, but without amusement, because it requires so very many words.

Thus the expert insists on getting what he must know, emphasizing the fact that without the information it is impossible for him to guess what sort of person his client is, or to know what ails him. This applies, with certain changes in phrase, to interviews for the purpose of deciding whether a person should or should not be employed, should or should not be fired, can or cannot perform this or that, and so on. The expert is entitled to the relevant and significant data, and he therefore sets out to get it. If there is any great difficulty, he explains how necessary it is to have the information, and when that is made fairly clear, then he inquires why in the world he can't get it.

Sometimes difficulties in living are illuminated at that very point. For example, in paranoid states there is the utmost secrecy about all sorts of things which, so far as I know, are of no interest to anybody but the patient. The psychiatrist, in trying to get at various things that he needs to know, may bump into these areas of secrecy; in such circumstances he may say, for example, "Am I to understand the difficulty that you have with this troublesome neighbor of yours without any information at all about it?" At this the patient may glare for a while, being in somewhat of a dilemma, because, as far as he is concerned, the psychiatrist really should be able to do just that; yet it *does* sound rather peculiar when put that way. If then the psychiatrist says, "Or is it some secret that you don't want to confess?" he may draw himself up, really indignant at this point, and say, "Well, I think that these things are not at all improved by discussion." Now that helps to make it very clear that the psychiatrist cannot be useful to him, and so the psychiatrist simply comments on that. Thus it becomes fairly evident that there are some very remarkable secrets in this person's life, secret even from him.

The interviewer is also entitled to exercise his skill in discouraging trivia, irrelevancies, graceful gestures for his amusement, and repetitions of things he has heard. It is perhaps harder for the younger interviewer to demonstrate his expertness in this respect than it is for him to insist on the data he must have. But if you are an expert in interpersonal relations, you are likely, for good reason, to doubt that you have too much lifetime ahead of you, and therefore you want to utilize it as well as you can. It is also profoundly impressive to people, in the lucid interval after they leave you, to realize that you have kept them to something that made sense, and that when they started telling you a thing all over again, you said, "Yes, yes. Now we want to inquire into so-and-so." In other words, the expert does not permit people to tell him things so beside the point that only God could guess how they happened to get into the account. And so from his first meeting with the patient until the end or interruption of an interview or series of interviews, the psychiatrist handles himself like an expert in interpersonal relations who is genuinely interested in the problems of the patient. He is careful to get all the details necessary to avoid misunderstanding and to clarify erroneous impressions unintentionally given by the patient, yet he is chary of encouragement toward any repetitive, circumstantial, or inconsequential detail in the report and comment of the patient. There is no time to spare in a psychiatric interview. If he sees that the patient is repeating himself, going into circumstances which are in no sense illuminating, or wandering into inconsequentialities about some fourth, fifth, or sixth removed person, he may, without unkindness, discourage such moves, tolerating only a minimum of wasted time, since he knows that there is plenty to do. Actually this is a kindness to the patient, for it communicates to him that the psychiatrist seems to know what he is doing, and with such hope in mind he will put up very nicely with what the psychiatrist does.

The psychiatrist also foregoes the satisfaction of any curiosity about matters into which there is no technical reason to inquire. He foregoes this in a *passive* fashion, in that he does not ask, for example, what particular fore-pleasures the person has learned in intercourse with his wife or sweetheart, when that is of no moment; moreover, he foregoes it very *actively*, by cutting off accounts when he has heard what is important, even though it would be thrilling to hear the rest. Again, the patient greatly appreciates this. First, he is spared the perhaps marked embarrassment of going into harrowing detail. Second, he realizes, even if only after he leaves the office, that "This doctor was trying to find out what *ailed* me. He wasn't trying to amuse himself." Such a discovery goes a long way in making for the durable benefit which I wish to come from a psychiatric interview. Patients are really immensely pleased to learn that the doctor can end matters when he gets what he wants to know, and that he can then turn his curiosity off and apply it to something else that really matters.

PSYCHIATRIC BANALITIES

Still another thing that the interviewer should eschew is all meaningless comment and clouding of issues. At the same time, he avoids giving tacit consent, by absence of comment, to delusion or grievous errors expressed by the patient—a point which

I shall discuss later. We often fail to realize just how meaningless many comments are. A lot of bromides from the culture and psychiatric banalities are handed out with the utmost facility, but I defy anyone to determine what most of them mean. For example, people refer to a "mother-fixation"—and when this is done by a psychiatrist in the course of a psychiatric interview, I think it deserves nothing short of a spanking. I grew up in the psychoanalytic school, and in studying schizophrenics—males only, after I found that I couldn't study female schizophrenics without getting more puzzled than they were—I discovered many mother-fixations. That is, I listened to a number of accounts of people's relationships with their mothers, but these were in every case accompanied by a wealth of detail which made of the relationship something which could never be appropriately and meaningfully condensed under the rubric, "mother-fixation." Nor could such a term be meaningful to any of these patients, who experienced their mothers in a great many ways, both devastating and wonderful. In other words, "mother-fixation" may be a beautiful abstract idea, useful for the psychiatrist's private ruminations; but to the person who suffers the "mother-fixation," the term is as nearly devoid of meaning, as near to being claptrap, as anything I can think of. Thus the psychiatrist tries to avoid meaningless comments and psychiatric banalities that prevent both his and the patient's learning anything, and merely give the patient a vague feeling that, "My God, I must have been terribly stupid; of course, that must be so, but why didn't I think of it?" In such a situation, there was nothing simply and usefully clear in what the psychiatrist said; he merely clouded the issue.

Thus, insofar as it is possible—and all of us fail now and then when one of our private interests is touched upon—the psychiatrist remembers that his role is that of an expert. He tries to keep to this role, no matter what attractive cul-de-sacs the patient may open up to him; if he does take an interest in the interview other than that of a person who is very hard at work in the most difficult of all labors—namely, understanding who somebody else is, what ails him, and what one can do that will be wise and durable in its results—he recognizes it and regrets it. From beginning to end, to the best of his ability, the psychiatrist tries to avoid being involved as a person—even as a dear and wonderful person—and keeps to the business of being an *expert*; that is, he remains one who, theoretically and in fact, deals with his patients only because he (the psychiatrist) has had the advantage of certain unique training and experience which make him able to help them.

In all this, the psychiatrist eschews with the greatest care all procedure which is calculated chiefly to impress the patient, to show that the psychiatrist is clairvoyant, or that he is possessed of omniscience. A psychiatrist, or any other expert interviewer, should have developed a certain humility, so that he may not be too inclined to act as if he knew all and his mind penetrated all, at a glance. He may feel that interviewing is hard work, as I recommend everyone should. It is, beyond perchance, very hard work.

Cultural Handicaps to the Work of the Psychiatrist

In the expert-client relationship with the patient, some of the extraordinary difficulties which the psychiatrist encounters in being expert arise from what may be called "antipsychiatric" elements in the culture itself—that is, elements in the culture which make the performance of psychiatric expertness far more difficult than is the demonstration of expertness in a great many other fields. Under this topic I could discuss a great many cultural attitudes that have been conspicuous throughout historic time, but I shall attempt to generalize only a few of those that constantly harass the psychiatric expert, just as they have always harassed people of Western European culture. First, in attempting to be psychiatric experts, we are very much afflicted by the fact that all people are taught that they *ought not* to need help, so that they are ashamed of needing it or feel that they are foolish to seek it or to expect it. And along with this, they come for psychiatric assistance with curious expectations as to what they are going to get, perhaps partly because this is so necessary to prop up self-esteem.

Second—and this is very widespread in the cultural heritage, so that people are taught it quite generally—is the belief that they should "know themselves," know what a fixed something-or-other called "human nature" is, know "right from wrong," and "good from bad," and be able to see through others in respect to all these important matters.

And third, people are more or less taught that they should be governed by "logic," or have "good sense"; or if they can't claim particularly good sense, then at least they should have "good natural instincts" and "good intuition," which ought to govern them in choosing the "right" way to act and to think about themselves and others.

Another idea which is very generally ingrained in personality is that one should be ashamed if one has not risen above and overcome the limitations of one's past, one's misfortunes, and one's mistakes; or if one hasn't, then one should occupy oneself with producing a very rich crop of verbalisms to show why, in spite of one's fineness and so on, these misfortunes were too much to be risen above and overcome.

Finally, as a sort of generalization of all of these, or in some people as yet another and separate antipsychiatric view: one should be independent. One should have no need for anyone else to tell one what to do or how to live. It was the culturally endorsed notion of independence which made the story of Robinson Crusoe so attractive in our unhappy youth—and a more recent demonstration of this notion appeared in a book which set up as the ideal of human maturity that one should be dependent only when sick, which I hope I have made clear is a somewhat dubious idea.

The Use of Methodic Procedure for Overcoming Personal Handicaps

The psychiatrist encounters extraordinary difficulties in being expert, not only because of these very widely spread antipsychiatric attitudes in the culture, but also because of inadequacies of his technical information. At the present stage of psychiatric knowledge, that is inevitable, because we do not yet grasp enough of the processes making up interpersonal relations to be adequate to all of the problems that arise in the course of our attempting to be psychiatrists. In addition, there is in all cases some measure of handicap arising from the psychiatrist's ignorance of interpersonal factors, which interferes with or precludes his participating as an expert in certain phases of the doctor-patient relationship. Now this may be a recurrent handicap in every one of his doctor-patient relationships, or practically every one—in which case one strongly surmises that the ignorance of interpersonal factors pertains primarily to the psychiatrist's grasp on himself. Or the handicap may vary from one of his doctor-patient relationships to another—in which case the handicap primarily pertains to characteristics of particular patients which the psychiatrist, because of his particular background and training, is unable to note, to observe.

None of us, with reasonable humility about the incompleteness of psychiatry and of our personal orientation, can expect to escape such handicaps. Therefore, in order to reduce the chances of serious difficulties arising from our ignoring or overlooking interpersonal processes in the psychiatric doctor-patient relationship, it is wise to make use, practically to the point of habituation, of a more or less methodic procedure for developing these relations with patients. While I cannot tell other psychiatrists just what procedure will be ideally suited to them, still there are some gross outlines which probably would be useful to practically anyone who does interviewing. Therefore I want to discuss a sort of diagram of method—or a diagram of the way in which one can develop methods for handling psychiatric interviews. By unobtrusively following such a method of procedure, the psychiatrist both saves time and demonstrates skill.

The psychiatric interview may be considered as made up of a series of stages which, while really hypothetical, fictional, abstract, and artificial, can be very useful for the psychiatrist to have in mind in arranging his time with the patient. More important, I believe that they are quite necessary for the achievement of the purpose of an intensive relationship of this kind. These stages are: first, the formal inception; second, the reconnaissance; third, the detailed inquiry; and fourth, the termination.

I shall discuss these stages in considerable detail later on, and for the moment shall outline only very briefly what I mean by them. The *inception* includes the formal reception of the person who comes to be interviewed and an inquiry about, or reference to, the circumstances of his coming. It should also include a brief, but considered, reference by the psychiatrist to any information already at his disposal; this is important not only to promote a feeling of confidence on the part of the patient, in the interviewer's straightforwardness, but also to provide an opportunity for the patient to amend the presumptive data which the psychiatrist may have received from another source, if necessary. Finally, an adequate reason for the conference must be established; that is, the psychiatrist should obtain adequate justification for the use of his skill.

Throughout this stage of the interview, the psychiatrist must remember that the person who consults him is a stranger—even though in other circumstances he may be an old friend. Thus the psychiatrist cannot know what impression anything that he says or does may make on this stranger, for he knows nothing of his background and nothing of the parataxic elements which may be very powerful in influencing his impressions. The psychiatrist must, therefore, be very alert to learn something of the impression that he and certain of his performances give, and at the same time very alert to learn how he himself is affected by certain things that the stranger may do and say. The interviewer should proceed in such a way that no complicating situation develops in this stage, for the inception of the interview may either greatly accelerate the achievement of the result desired or make that result practically unattainable.

The second step in procedure, the *reconnaissance*, which should be initiated as "naturally" as possible, consists in obtaining a rough outline of the social or personal history of the patient. In this stage, the interviewer is concerned with trying to get some notion of the person's identity—who he is and how he happened to get to be the person who has come to the office. Thus the interviewer asks conventional questions about age, order of siblings, date of marriage, and so on; he does not try to develop a psychiatric history, but tries to orient himself as to certain basic probabilities. The skill of the interviewer in obtaining and interpreting this history may often largely determine the ease or difficulty of the succeeding detailed inquiry. Moreover, the time to be spent in achieving the purpose of the interview or series of interviews may depend on the concise accuracy with which this history is obtained.

The next stage, the *detailed inquiry*, depends considerably, although not exclusively, on the ostensible purpose of the interview—a topic which I shall discuss shortly. The larger part of these lectures will deal with the principles and techniques of the detailed inquiry—that is, with some of the particulars that make up the almost unlimited variety of subtleties and complexities of this long stretch of inquiry into another person's life and problems. For the moment, I will say only that while the interviewer is governed in this inquiry by the ostensible purpose of the interview, he never carries out a good interview if he forgets what it is really for—namely, to permit an expert in human relations to contribute something to another person's success in living.

The fourth step of the interview, in this particular abstract scheme, is either the *termination* or the *interruption* of the psychiatric interview. By termination, I mean that the interviewer does not expect to see the person again; he is through. And by interruption, I mean that the interviewer has seen his client as long as he is going to on that particular day, and will see him again on the next day, or at some future date. If the interview is interrupted, the psychiatrist should give the patient a prescription for the interval, as a setting for the next session— for example, he may suggest something that the patient might try to recall. If the interview is terminated, the interviewer should make a final statement. In general, the main purpose to be attained, either in terminating an interview or in interrupting it for any length of time, is the consolidation of what has been achieved in terms of some durable benefit for the interviewee.

CHAPTER
III

Some General Technical
Considerations in Interviewing

Types of Psychiatric Interviews

BEFORE I DISCUSS the stages of the psychiatric interview in detail, I would like to mention several considerations which affect the course of the interview as a whole, and which affect the detailed inquiry in particular. One is the ostensible purpose of the interview. If the interview is for the purpose of finding out whether there is an adequate reason for firing a person whom somebody wants fired, naturally the interviewer does not cover all of the same topics that he would cover if he were attempting to discover, for example, why the person has precocious ejaculation in all of his attempts to establish his heterosexual prowess. Thus the interviewer is governed by the ostensible purpose of the interview; yet the assumptions I have named are not changed, and the attempt of the interviewer to be of some use to the person cannot be yielded, for this is the reason why the person does reveal what the interviewer needs to know.

To give some idea of the formal spread of ostensible purposes in psychiatric interviews, let me mention, first, the consultation carried out for purposes of diagnosis with a view to advising and perhaps facilitating the securing of competent treatment elsewhere. That is, the psychiatrist tries to determine the nature of the interviewee's personal difficulties in living, and to advise him with whom, and in what way, treatment or benefit may be obtained. Even though the interviewer in this case does not himself contemplate undertaking intensive treatment of the patient, he still must accomplish a good deal therapeutically, in the broad sense that I have spoken of; the patient may not be able even to reveal many of his greatest difficulties in living unless it becomes evident that this doctor will be useful in encouraging him to survive them for the time being, at least.

Then there is the interview which is, in fact, the initial conference in either brief psychotherapy or a potential continued-treatment situation; that is, the interviewer undertakes both diagnosis and the establishment of a professional acquaintance with a view to carrying on treatment himself.

These two are very different matters. In the former type of psychiatric consultation, it is a foregone conclusion that unless the patient proves to be charming beyond his wildest dreams, this particular doctor will simply tell him where to get treatment. I think that that is a distinctly easier job than the interview in which the psychiatrist not only finds out, it is hoped, some of the major ailments of the patient, but also communicates to him the conviction, which the psychiatrist himself shares, that he can aid the patient in getting rid of them. The element of the future relationship so strongly colors some interviews of the latter type that I have known psychiatrists to overlook what ailed the patient in the process of arranging to treat him, as a result of which the treatment was somewhat difficult. On the other hand, when it is a foregone conclusion that this particular interviewer will perform no miracles, but will just tell the patient where to go and why, getting the necessary data is greatly facilitated.

The next type of interview I wish to mention is held again for the purpose of diagnosing a difficulty in living, but with an emphasis on influencing the environment rather than the patient. For example, wives sometimes come to discuss treatment for their husbands, or ladies their sweethearts, or vice versa, with the idea that this might take some kinks out of the relationship. For all I know, it sometimes does. Schoolteachers sometimes come to discuss getting treatment for difficult children, with the idea that this might make it easier to live and

teach in the same room with them. And clergymen have been
known to feel that they needed a little technical knowledge
about their relations with communicants. Parents, custodians
of jails, judges, and very intelligent members of law firms sometimes wonder if a little technical advice about the mental
health and probable needs of their clients might not be an aid
in helping them. In such cases, the psychiatrist is supposed to
produce the benefit, so far as the given situation is concerned,
by some effect through other people, or institutions, or something of that kind. That does not suspend the necessity for also
helping the person who comes to the interview, if the interviewer is really to get the data he needs; it does not forbid
that something should be done for this person to help him to
live.

There is also an increasing field of interviewing in connection with industrial or commercial personnel management.
Thus the psychiatrist may be asked to interview a prospective
promotee or transferee for some organization which has an en-
lightened official who thinks that there is something to be
gained from the study of personality. Or if a person repeatedly
fails to show up for work because of ill-health, he may be
advised to see the psychiatrist; such procedures are becoming
accepted in the growing field of industrial medicine. Incidentally, there seem to be an increasing number of major gen-
erals in the British, American, and doubtless the Russian armies,
who have already discovered that the company commander
who gets somewhat acquainted with his troops—the one who
might say, "You look sort of down-in-the-mouth today, Joe.
What's the trouble? Bad news from home?" and hears in return
something like, "Well, I think my girl has fallen for somebody
else," and then talks to him a little—is the commander whose
company has very few absences without leave, and a strikingly
small proportion of acute psychoneurotic disturbances under
fire, and so on. In other words, it is beginning to be clear in
many places that a great deal of the seeming difficulty in the
productiveness of people is related to obscure problems away
from the job—in the home, in the community, in the church, or

elsewhere—and that it can be very useful to have someone around who is not too free with advice but who can be fairly skillful at finding out what the person is really worrying about, so that he can say, "Well, isn't this or that probable, and can't you brace yourself for one or the other of them?" Such an apparently simple thing as that has an immensely useful effect on these apparent difficulties in management–labor relations, commissioned officer–enlisted man relations, and various other types of elaborately organized interpersonal cooperation.

As I have said, the ostensible purpose of the interview has a good deal to do with the exact procedure, but nevertheless it is fundamental that the interviewer convey to the interviewee more feeling of capacity, of adequacy to go on living, and of doing perhaps better as a result of the conference—even, for example, in a case where the interviewee may get fired as a consequence of his and the interviewer's finding that he is really greatly handicapped for dealing with the particular organization in which he happens to be. It is not enough that the interviewer should find out something and give a really convincing demonstration of it. The interviewee must also get something out of it.

The Use of Transitions in Interviewing

The topic of transitions is of such peculiar significance in connection with the whole procedure of the interview that I want to discuss it before proceeding any further. Although the making of transitions is strikingly important in the detailed inquiry, it is a necesary part of the technique of interviewing at every stage. And it is so peculiarly an abstraction of technique that it has nothing to do with the ostensible purpose, but is worth while for the interviewer to have organized in his mind no matter on what basis he interviews another person.

When I talk about how to make transitions, I simply mean how to move about in the interview. It is imperative, if you want to know where you are with another person, that you proceed along a path that he can at least dimly follow, so that he doesn't get lost completely as to what you are driving at. When he gets lost, very often you do too, and one or the other of you may not know it. The law of diminishing returns then begins to operate with great vigor without the patient's quite realizing it—and often without the psychiatrist's quite realizing it. It is ideal, if you can, to go step by step, with sufficient waving of signal flags and so on, so that there is always something approaching a consensus as to what is being discussed. Unfortunately, with many people that would mean that you would have to live several months with them; and so, when you are conducting a psychiatric interview, you may need to vary from this idea of always proceeding toward a goal which is unknown but can nonetheless be designated so that the patient can see what you are driving at. Actually, the interviewer must change directions quite frequently. He chokes off topics which, although they interest the patient, he identifies as improbably useful—that is, as taking vastly more time than any probable utility will justify. He must ask about some things which the patient is very skillful at eluding, and, as a result, the interview must sometimes move from one obscure situation to another, with the interviewer not always being certain that the patient knows just what he is asking about or certain that he understands exactly what the patient is trying to say.

I look upon transitions in interviews as one of the very important technical details that ought always to get considerable attention, requiring a sort of quiet, continuing alertness in all your work in dealing with strangers in a serious and intimate fashion. Notice that when you speak of changing the subject—that's one way of putting it—it doesn't tell the whole story. There are people who, I believe, have never stayed on the same subject for two consecutive remarks. And there are interviewers who seem to do little better. It is very easy to move from what you were discussing to something else that has popped into your mind; and if you do that without noticing what you have done, it is quite possible that you may obtain the most fantastic ideas of your interviewee. Thus it is always well to notice—with the same ease with which people can notice such a world of things that are going on without losing their place—when you change the subject. The changing of the subject can very well be treated in one of at least three ways, which are important and are by no means artificial abstractions.

The first of these we may call the *smooth transition*. When the interviewer wishes to change the subject, he can make the transition by a more or less adequate, and at least superficially truthful, statement which definitely says, in effect, "Well, now, that brings up the topic of so-and-so. Eh?" The patient might wear himself out trying to guess how it brought it up, but at least the interviewer has taken him by the hand and led him to the new topic. There are a good many times when the interviewer may use some little comment such as, "Oh, yes, well, sometimes that's due to so-and-so. I wonder if by any chance you've had experience of that kind?" In other words, he moves from one thing to another quite smoothly, so that the other person feels that this is really a very clear, collaborative inquiry. Now, an interviewer is not apt to do that if he does not realize that he is going to change the subject. And if he doesn't realize such things, he may lose his client.

In the *accentuated* or *accented transition* you do not use one of these polite ways of moving yourself and the patient hand in hand from one topic to another, but you rustle your feathers, as it were, and somehow indicate that, "Well, the world is about to undergo some mild change." In my case I usually begin to growl, rather like a ball bearing with some sand in it, just to indicate that something is about to happen. I want to drop what is going on, emphatically; not in such a way that it is forgotten forever, but with such emphasis as to disturb the set, as the old experimental psychologists might call it. I want that which has been discussed not to influence that which is now to be discussed. Suppose the person has just been showing me what an unutterably lovely soul he has. I will then sort of growl a bit as a preliminary to saying something like, "With what sort of person do you find yourself really hateful?" As a matter of fact, I probably wouldn't do anything quite that crude. But the point is that as long as he is full of the idea of convincing me of his beautiful soul, it would really be uncouth for me to proceed smoothly to attempt to find out how the devil he is a nuisance. But with the accented change, he may forget what he was talking about. People are apt to get a little insecure, you know, when it is suggested that the weather is going to change, and the predictions aren't dependable. In any case it causes a little pause, a sort of empty pause, which is not being smoothly, socially conversational. And then, without commotion—without startling the patient—I introduce the new topic. In this way the later data is not poisoned by the exploration that was in progress before, as it might be with a smooth transition.

Then there is the *abrupt transition*, at which, I am sorry to say, many interviewers seem to be past masters—and I should not wish to encourage them to improve their art. Nevertheless, it has its uses. I am not, however, suggesting a transition so abrupt that the patient is suddenly so startled that he can't guess what on earth the interviewer has said. I mean, rather, that a new topic is introduced which has relevance, but which is introduced at what would be described as a socially awkward point, and without warning. This sort of thing may be done to avoid, or to provoke, anxiety. I may say here that many an interview passes from the informative to the nebulous because the patient has become acutely anxious; but, on the other hand, some interviews would never get to be psychiatric interviews if the patient were not made anxious. The question relates to the way in which the patient is made anxious. It is properly done when the patient is taken through an upsetting period to definitely reassuring material, or from something that was going on with greatly increasing risk to the situation to something which is remarkably reassuring.

To sum up, the smooth transition is used to move gently to a new topic; the accented transition saves time and clarifies the situation; and the abrupt transition is ordinarily used either to avoid dangerous anxiety or to provoke anxiety where you can't get anywhere otherwise.

The Taking of Notes During the Interview

I am often asked my opinion about the making of written notes during the course of the interview, considered from the point of view of its effect on the psychiatrist and on the patient. There is a great variation among people in the degree to which certain behavior is automatic; and so there may be people so expert at shorthand that they can jot down rather automatically a great deal of what they are listening to and still leave the field of awareness free to participate in the work of the interview, and there may even be people who can make longhand notes which are useful to them later without particularly occupying their attention during the actual session. The only times that I have ever made notes during an interview with the feeling that it did not seriously interfere with the work that I had to do was when I dealt with people whose production rate was very low—certain puzzled schizophrenics, and one patient with a serious disorder in the region between schizophrenia and the obsessional illnesses. Schizophrenic patients have great difficulty in completing their sentences, often losing their place before they are through with a sentence, and they speak relatively infrequently, spending a good deal of time in starting and stopping. Since I was greatly interested theoretically in what the disorder of thought and speech was, I did take down quite completely a great many of my hours with a few puzzled schizophrenics. In fact, I had one patient who talked so slowly and had such a theoretically very important condition that I wrote down verbatim what he said. Unhappily, I fear that this record will not become available to posterity, because I can't translate my writing without taking two or three times as much time as it took to conduct the interviews. That, in its way, tells a story: the fact that I was not paying enough attention to write legibly suggests that I was busy with something else. And the obverse of that is more or less my opinion about taking notes: if enough attention is paid to them so they are legible, this is very apt indeed to interfere with things of much greater importance to the patient, if not to the psychiatrist.

The psychiatric interviewer is supposed to be doing three things: considering what the patient could mean by what he says; considering how he himself can best phrase what he wishes to communicate to the patient; and, at the same time, observing the general pattern of the events being communicated or discussed. In addition to that, to make notes which will be of more than evocative value, or come anywhere near being a verbatim record of what is said, in my opinion is beyond the capacity of most human beings.

Even if the interviewer were able to do all this, when he deals with patients who are quite suspicious, even paranoid, in their attitudes, the making of notes will probably guarantee that the interviewer hears an exceedingly studied group of communications, in which all the nuances which he might otherwise catch on to are missing. Nevertheless, there are occasions—for example, when I am getting the gross social data about a person—when I do feel that I should have a few notes. On such occasions I tell the patient that I have really a gift for forgetting things that might be handy, and therefore, if he doesn't mind, I shall make a few notes as to the number of siblings and one thing and another. At other times, however, when I have felt that something of great importance could be obtained from an interview, I have taken considerable pains to see that the recording of the interview was entirely exterior to the patient's awareness.

In the interrogation of patients before staff conferences, the patient is not only in the presence of a shorthand reporter, but also of a large number of psychiatrists. Many psychiatrists consider this a relatively barbarous practice, but since I found it in existence at several places where I worked, I put it to such use as I could. I think that the fact that a record is being made is initially quite distressing to many of the patients, but there are so many other things that are distressing about the interrogation that most of the patients, I think, forget that a record is being made before the session is over. Nevertheless, the reporting does not facilitate communication.

To put the whole thing succinctly, I think that most psychiatrists, if they are really engaged in conducting and understanding a psychiatric interview, are too busy to have much time to make written notes, even if making notes did not have a distinctly estopping effect on the patient. I think that patients, like the rest of us, can usually talk with relative freedom if only their own and the other fellow's memories are later to be consulted as to what was said. All of us become considerably more cautious if there is to be a written record of it. I myself can, through long experience, talk in the presence of a recording machine; I am able to be more interested in whether or not I have gotten across what I am trying to present than preoccupied with the inhibiting effect of the recording machinery. Yet if I knew that a stranger was going to take over the record before I had a chance to look at it, I might feel differently about it—in spite of the fact that I have considerable faith in saying what I mean, aside from minor accidents in speaking, and fatigue that sometimes prevents me from finding the words I am looking for. These are advantages rarely possessed by a person undergoing a psychiatric interview; even if in his better moments he feels quite able to speak the language, the psychiatric interview is a situation of considerable stress, in which he is likely to feel at a disadvantage, and the idea that a record is being made increases his disadvantage still more.

A verbatim record of an interview, until it has been heavily annotated, is almost invariably remarkably misleading. I have had some recordings of interviews which I have regarded as astonishingly good teaching material, but when I have sprung these on intelligent colleagues, I have often found them barking up trees that I hadn't seen—if, indeed, such trees were ever there, and I came to realize that they weren't. In other words, the complete meaning of a conversation is not to be found in the verbatim verbal context of the communication, but is reflected in all sorts of subtle interplay. For example, very slight changes of tone suggesting the faintest hint of irritation on the part of the psychiatrist often switch the patient from an attempt at concealment to a very reasonable compromise between what he thinks it is safe to tell and what the facts may have been. Such things do not appear in the most perfect verbal record. Thus, to give a third person a notion of all that happened in an interview, one would have to annotate the written record by adding the impressions that went with different statements, explaining why things were put as they were, and so on; only in this way could the richness of the interchange in a two-centered unitary situation begin to be apparent.

The Interpersonal Integration of the Interviewer and Interviewee

I would now like to review some of the things that I have said from a somewhat different standpoint. What I have said about the course of the interview through its various stages and the transition during the interview from topic to topic may be seen to imply the beginning, course, and termination of an interpersonal situation. Psychiatry studies interpersonal relations, which occur only in interpersonal situations; such situations imply something more than the presence of two people somewhere; they concern two people who are *involved* with each other—and that we call *integration*. Further, an interpersonal situation, of which the interview situation is a particular instance, is integrated by—brought into being by, held together by, and the course of its events, to a certain extent, determined by—something in the two people concerned which is *reciprocal*, and the manifestations of which coincide approximately in time. Thus one may say that the interview situation, or series of situations, is *integrated by coincident reciprocal motivation* of interviewee and interviewer.

A great deal about the psychiatric interview can be learned if we consider it from the standpoint of the reasons for its occurrence—that is, if we examine the reciprocal motivation that coincides in a particular interview. From what we know about the integration of interpersonal situations I derive the statement which I have already emphasized so much: an interview must promise to be of some use to the interviewee; he feels entitled to, and should have, some gain from it. If his expectation is in no way met, the interviewer will not have much of an idea of what is going on. Thus, no matter how apparently inferior, or unfortunate, or needy, or what not, another human being may be, the interviewer must realize that his profit from the interview must be more than imaginary. He must have a sufficient motive for going on with it; otherwise, even though he may sound as if he were really answering the interviewer's questions, he will actually be doing something different.

As an expert in the participant observation of interpersonal situations, the interviewer has the task of so influencing the interview situation that the closely observed course of his participation will reveal the major handicaps and major advantages in living which are relatively durable characteristics of the interviewee. Now, that is a very big requirement, and my experience suggests to me that many of us, having discovered a *few* of the patient's handicaps, may use a very lively imagination to provide us with something like a comprehensive picture of him as a person. The need to do that is understandable, but the practice yields distorted data. Of course, the inconspicuous intervention of the psychiatrist will not serve to reveal all of the patient's reasonably probable handicaps and assets fully, and will not result in their being documented or proved; some of them will be indicated only. But they should not be entirely overlooked or left to the interviewer's imagination in retrospect when he is writing his report.

It is the interpersonal events and the pattern of their course which generate the data of the interview; that is, the interviewer experiences the ways in which the interpersonal events follow each other, what seeming relationships they have to one another, what striking inconsistencies occur, and so on. Thus the data of the interview may come, not so much from the answers to questions, but from the timing and stress of what was said, the slight misunderstandings here and there, the occasions when the interviewee got off the subject, perhaps volunteering very important facts which had not been asked for, and so on. And so as an interviewer grows more skillful, he realizes with increasing clarity that what he must do is to watch the course of events and observe how they, as a pattern of progression, give rise to a very wide field of data about the other person with whom he is concerned. His use of this data, and his skill in drawing inferences from it, will grow with experience. Yet, until he has the information to be gained from this kind of participant observation, he has nothing with which to begin; and it cannot be obtained by the charmingly simple procedure of sitting at a desk and, with a feeling of utterly detached isolation from the person out in front, shooting questions at him, and perhaps checking his answers on a form.

The all but inevitable extreme obscurity of the events early in the interview, and the continuing complexity of so many of those events making up its course, make it useful to be unobtrusively methodical, as well as constantly alert. In other words, the interviewer is quite clearly aware of the type of significant data that he may reasonably expect in different phases of the interview; he takes steps to secure these data; he validates, or marks for subsequent validation, anything which seems needlessly indefinite or improbable; and he notes most carefully any occasion when material reasonably to be expected *has not* come forth. All this implies what I have already stressed—the advisability of very methodically, although unobtrusively, including in each interview the four phases which I have mentioned, and of accomplishing in the formal initiation of the interview certain very definite steps. Because of the sometimes impossible complexity of relations with a comparatively unknown other person, it is wise for the interviewer to ingrain in himself an outline of the ways in which these steps can be taken, developing patterns of action which will work so effectively and so unnoticed that he will not have to take time out to consider what the next step is to be.

But since no outline can possibly anticipate the variations that may occur in a personal relationship with a stranger, it is not enough that the interviewer knows just what he expects to do; he must also be alert for any suggestion that something has happened which is unexpected, because the *novelties* which occur in an inconspicuously methodical investigation are the things that distinguish its results. For example, among the most significant characteristics in the course of events making up an interview are the absences of those events which all or most of the interviewer's previous experience leads him to expect. A person may build up a course of historic data which, in the interviewer's experience, has always meant that certain events would follow. When this sequence does not appear in a particular patient's account, the interviewer does not necessarily get excited about it, but he does not overlook the omission. The fact that the data reasonably to be expected from a certain movement in an interview have not appeared *may* be highly revealing, and, in any case, is far too promising a matter to be overlooked or forgotten.

Somewhat similarly, the psychiatrist notices any points at which the patient seems to have no grasp on things which the psychiatrist regards as necessary or important in life, or in the patient's work. At such points, instead of concluding that he is dealing with someone stupid, the psychiatrist offers some hints as to what the information might be, to determine if it actually is lacking. If it is, he may offer some comment which is as simple, unassuming, and clear as he can make it, to see what happens, because there are a good many people who require only a hint to catch on to long streams of implications, and it is very useful to discover that.

Or, as another example, the psychiatrist may be puzzled by something the patient says. This does not always justify the interviewer in immediately jumping into the situation and asking about it; there are times when it is very wise to wait to resolve any puzzle or doubts. However, if events have not been made clear at some particular point, the interviewer should *know* that such is the case, so that when there seems to be an opportunity for a perfectly good transition, or when nothing in particular seems to be going on and the patient is waiting for questions, he can bring this point up again and indicate that he is in doubt as to the precise meaning. People very quickly come to understand that what they have said may not communicate perfectly to the listener, and they are quite reasonable about illustrating the various conclusions that they have stated.

Now, observing all these things is a function of the interviewer's *alertness*. No matter how smoothly things are going, he must be alert for something new or unexpected. Alertness is a function that is in a sense intimately related to that type of activity which people call "thought," but which is actually vastly more extensive than that which we know as "thought." For more precise purposes we may apply to this activity the term "covert process"—something that cannot be observed, but only inferred—which is in contrast to the other type of referential operations, the *overt*, which can be observed, although sometimes only by the initiate. Some may say that covert processes can be observed by introspection. Doubtless some covert processes could be observed this way, were it not that the process of introspection is apt to destroy the clarity of the covert process. In any case, the field of covert processes concerned in human behavior is vastly wider than anything that anyone has ever discovered by introspection.

Since one's alertness is a *function of covert processes*, it is useful in training for interviewing to have in mind the genera of data to be expected from phase to phase in the interview. That can be put, if you please, as "knowing what you are looking for"; however, I hesitate to describe it that way, for anyone who thinks in such terms is in very serious danger of believing that he looks from an isolated observing standpoint on performances to which he is related solely as an observer, and this the interviewer cannot do. There are no psychiatric data that can be observed from a detached position by a person in no way involved in the operation. All psychiatric data arise from participation in the situation that is observed—in other words, by participant observation. Thus, instead of "knowing what one is looking for," one wants to be *alert to the possibilities of the immediate future of the relationship in which one is involved*. This is why I cannot say, "Here are seventeen tables of events that can characterize interviews; now, you memorize all these and then you will always know just what to expect." No such thing is possible.

Alertness can never be brought about in a useful fashion solely in response to things that can be precisely communicated in words, unless the communication is of a peculiarly extraordinary character. Of course, if without warning I look wildly toward the door and shout, "Fire!" I do use a word, and the hearer's alertness would be very powerfully influenced by that communication. But that is most exceptional, and even so, it is scarcely *verbal* communication. It is a queer kind of warning of great danger, very little different from the ringing of a very large gong. Thus I cannot teach anyone *what* to expect—what to be alert to so that he will not overlook important events. Instead I am attempting to encourage the organization of thought in a fashion that will include, in this very broad sense, the functions of the covert processes, a great many of which cannot be formulated accurately.

But, when I say that the psychiatrist must be greatly alert, I do not suggest that he uses this alertness simply in observing the *patient*, the *patient's* behavior, what the *patient* says, and so on. Instead, he is at all times conscious of the fact that this is a performance of *two* people, in which the patient's behavior and what he says are adjusted, to the best of the patient's information and ability, to what he guesses about the psychiatrist. Correspondingly, the psychiatrist's comments, questions, remarks, innuendoes, and so on are effective to the extent that he is aware of the patient's attitude toward him, and is aware of all that he has thus far learned of the patient's background, his experience, and what sort of a person he is. Thus the psychiatrist, insofar as it is possible, concentrates his attention on the processes going on between himself and the other person, or involving himself and the other person, and not on something as remote as, "What is this patient of mine doing and saying?" If, however, he should add, "with me and to me," then he begins to make sense.

CHAPTER
IV

The Early Stages of the
Interview

The Formal Inception

I WISH NOW to discuss rather fully, within the frame of reference I have tried to set up, the first of the four phases which I have mentioned: the *formal inception* of the interview, including the reception of the interviewee and the overt establishment of the type of interpersonal situation that is expected to ensue.

First, let us consider the actual "physical" encounter with the interviewee. He may be an utter stranger found unexpectedly sitting in one's waiting room, or he may be an old friend who disconcertingly converts himself, in the course of a commonplace conversation, into a client seeking expert advice. Or, of course, he may be someone who has made an appointment by telephone to see the psychiatrist. The way in which the interviewee is received can greatly accelerate the achievement of the result desired, or it can make the result practically unattainable. From the moment that the interviewer and interviewee first see each other, very important aspects of the psychiatric interview are in progress. And from this moment, the interviewer must realize that his own convenience, his own past malfeasances, and so on, are not anywhere near as important as the assumption that here is someone to be treated with respectful seriousness because he wants to be benefited, or at least can be benefited.

That means that the interviewer does not greet his patient—who may be both penetrating and hostile—with a lot of social hokum that might be all right in meeting aged maternal relatives. I think that the social manner of some doctors has antagonized a larger proportion of their really life-size patients than have their failures in skill and their obvious stupidities of judgment. Any person who notices what is going on is not amused at being treated simply as another statistical instance of a patient who must be made to feel comfortable, a procedure which some interviewers suppose they accomplish by treating the patient like an animated art object, or an imbecile, or something of the kind. Formal statements are perhaps not the ideal way to start psychiatric interviews; habitual utterances —especially those accompanied by the kind of handshake which reminds one who is sensitive of a curious relationship between what he has in his hand and a dead fish—are not conducive to establishing the claims to interpersonal expertness to which I have referred. And per contra, astonishing greetings such as, "Oh, *hello*, come in!" which might be all right with a person recently returned from London, are not useful substitutes.

May I suggest that a stranger is fully as bothered about meeting the interviewer as the interviewer would be in a similar situation. Thus while I don't try to show a great welcome to the patient, I do try to act as if he were expected—that is, I try to know the name of a person who makes an appointment to see me for the first time, and to greet him with it, relieving him of any morbid anxiety as to whether he came on the wrong day, and so on. And I suggest that he come in, which is a form of hospitality that extends to many branches of civilization, and is, in fact, I suppose, indispensable wherever there is a doctrine that a man's house, or office, is his castle. I take a good look at him while he is at the door, and after that I do not stare at him. Once he is in, I indicate where he should sit. I think most of us have experienced the relief, in a difficult situation, of having someone indicate where we may sit; it relieves us of all the wondering about where the other person intends to sit, where it is proper to sit, and so on. One experience of mine impressed this on me: A great man, who had invited me to confer with him about a paper, courteously asked me in, and then sat down and looked at me for a long time without asking me to be seated. I decided that that was a poor way to treat a stranger.

Next I tell the patient what I have learned so far as to why he is there. If he telephoned me to make the appointment, I may say, "I gathered from our conversation over the telephone that you have a problem of such-and-such a nature," putting a little question mark at the end. If I am aware that he is there because someone else sent him, I may say, "Doctor So-and-so," or the chief of the division, or what not, "sent you, I understand, for such-and-such reasons," again with a question mark. In other words, I show that I have paid attention to what little data have been presented to me—I have, for example, taken the trouble to notice what was said to me over the telephone. And I am straightforward to the extent of my data —and even though in certain special circumstances that is not true, at least I try to give the client something of my impression of why he is there. These first data are probably irrelevant; for instance, what he told me over the telephone may well have been merely an excuse for seeing me, or the boss' reason for sending the client may have represented a complete misapprehension on the boss' part. But by laying my cards on the table—insofar as is practicable—I give him, at the very beginning of things, a magnificent opportunity to correct the situation, to revise the information I so far have. Thus when I give him my impression of the story that I have either from him or from somebody else, he can react with anything from, "Yes, that's right, Doctor, and it's a great problem," all the way to, "What? Why I never dreamed of it. How is it possible for you to have such a misunderstanding?" In the latter case, I certainly don't say, "Well, that's the case." Instead, I say something like, "Well, now tell me what really *is* the case." And he begins to tell me. Thus the interviewer operates so that no complicating situation develops in this first meeting with the stranger.

In this way, it is easier for the patient to get started if he doesn't happen to be the person the interviewer thinks he is—and he usually isn't. He begins to feel, "Well, we've begun." And as a matter of fact, we have begun; something has gone on with the fewest possible words, and with the least vacant utterance and gesture. The end of this first stage comes when he has made some statement that I can assume gives him the feeling that he has transmitted to me some idea of his problem and of himself. But I don't try to *find out* at this stage what ails him, for, as I have already said, no one can understand what ails a person without knowing that person. But I try to let him feel that I do know something—that he has, at least, explained his presence. By that time we are ready for the second stage.

Since I have touched on the psychiatrist's use of collateral data—that is, information obtained from some source other than the patient himself—perhaps I should go into this further at this point. A question is sometimes raised as to whether the psychiatrist should receive such data. The problem, as I see it, is not so much one of whether he receives such data, but of what he does with it.

When very grave issues are concerned—for example, if the patient is seriously disordered, or fairly obviously in danger of serious mental disorder, and is confronted with the making of decisions that vastly transcend his ability, so that other people are badly worried about his having to make them—I would regard it as simply quixotic devotion to some curious doctrine for the psychiatrist not to avail himself of any information he can get that will bear on the problem concerned. But what he *does* with that information is often a very delicate problem of technique.

Whether the interviewer has sought out information from sources other than the patient, or whether it has been thrust upon him in the shape of a document that precedes the interviewee, or something of that kind, I have gradually come to feel that it is very important indeed to conduct the interview on the basis of that which is given *in the interview*. However, on some occasions I may use collateral data in unobtrusively directing the course of the interview.

For example, I may be asked to see a man who is applying for a certain government job because the chief of the bureau that is about to employ him feels very uncomfortable about him. From the bureau chief, I hear all sorts of things, including the fact that this man was once a patient in a mental hospital for two years, allegedly with a very serious mental disorder. In the course of the interview, I am able to inquire several times whether something that was being discussed ever got serious enough to be genuinely incapacitating. The answer in each case is, "Oh no! No indeed!" There is no suggestion that this man has ever had anything remotely like a mental disorder; the possibility is denied categorically, from every approach. Toward the close of the interview, I take counsel with myself and discover that I am not quite clear on his chronology of employment. I then say, "Now let's track down, year after year, just what you were doing and where." When he comes to the fatal years there is a pause, and things don't go so well. I say, "Well, you continued in your former employment through that year?" "No. No, I didn't." I wait for about thirty seconds, and then I say, "Well?" And he says, "As a matter of fact, I had some difficulty with my wife at that time, and had to take some time off from my employment. I was actually so upset by this business that I stopped work for a year and a half and took a trip." I say, "Well, well. Where did you go?" The man tells about the start of a trip, and then suddenly says, "Did you know that I was in a mental hospital?" To this I say, "For God's sake! Tell me about it." And he does.

I am pleased with that, because I would not have asked him about this. In this relationship, I have not told him in the beginning what I know, while he has become highly informative about many things that are both good and bad, from his standpoint—excepting that he has reserved something from me; I think he would go away feeling that he had been in the hands of a crook if I were to reveal in the end that I knew all about that something. The very thing that I insist is of vital importance in the psychiatric interview—namely, that the patient get something from it—would be endangered by his discovering that the cards had been stacked against him all the time. But, as a matter of fact, I don't know that very many people who reserve something from the doctor really feel, on sober second thought, that they have pulled the wool over the doctor's eyes. Many people who never overcome the inhibitions they set on themselves before coming to the interview wonder, in the two or three hours after they leave, whether they haven't been fools for not revealing the data which they suppressed. During the interview, they carefully protected this omission, this gap in the data, but because I have given them so many chances to fill it in, they can hardly help but notice in retrospect that it has appeared as a gap. It may then occur to the patient that such success in concealment has in it elements of personal failure.

This is an exception to what I have already stated: that in general, when a person meets me for the first time by order of, or recommendation of, someone else, I establish the situation as best I can by giving him, with as much frankness as I can, a very condensed outline of the highly significant things that I have been told or asked to determine, or what not. But in telling him this, I am chary with any rich detail, any possibly misleading emphasis, and so on, which the informant may have conveyed. I refrain from communicating any of the innuendo which is almost always present in a third person's talking about a second person, and I literally disadvise any interviewer's being very much influenced by such innuendo. It is not that those who send people to the interviewer intend to deceive him in advance; they simply don't know any better. Most people in referring somebody to a psychiatrist try to show that they know something about psychiatry—an innocent conceit, but one which is unfortunate if the psychiatrist enters into it.

Thus I tell the interviewee any presumably incontrovertible facts which have been laid before me, entirely minus any elements of interpretation by the person who communicated them to me. Telling the patient the gross facts as they have been given to me often saves a good deal of time. If what has been told me is not true, I want to hear the correction immediately.

In general, there is no reason in the world, so far as I know, for not letting the patient in on the facts as the psychiatrist was told them, *unless* some of them may be very disturbing. There is no reason to pronounce the patient insane as a preliminary to helping him regain his sanity. For example, the psychiatrist may be told so many disturbing things about a person that it seems practically a foregone conclusion that he has a serious mental disorder. But there is no sense in engaging in a prolonged psychiatric examination if the psychiatrist accepts all this as fact. In a great many years, I have rarely found the facts given to be literally facts. Even when the patient was fully as sick as had been indicated to me, the picture that I obtained in four, five, or six hours of inquiry was quite different from the picture I had been given in advance, and implied possibilities of treatment in the future which had not been implied by the information transmitted to me.

In general, collateral information should not be refused without good reason. However, when somebody very obscurely related to or probably hostile to the patient volunteers information, certainly one should discover the reason for this very "helpful" intervention before accepting it. For example, a husband may consult me because his wife is threatening divorce. In a couple of days the wife calls me, and wants to talk with me. It is a good idea to inquire what the lady has in mind: Does she feel the need of a psychiatrist for her own troubles, or what? No, she doesn't; she wants to tell me all about her husband. My general attitude in such cases is rather forbidding. For instance, I may say, "I should like very much to get the facts, but since I'm just beginning to understand your husband's difficulties, I do think we ought to wait a little while. I don't want to be unduly confused by too many facts all at once." Thus, when the interest of the informant is definitely hostile to the person with whom the interviewer is dealing, it pays to maintain a very judicious detachment in receiving this information and in venturing any comments on it; the interviewer is entitled to notice that the motivation for the action may not be constructive. That doesn't necessarily make the data bad, but it should inspire caution in the use of the data. And since it is very often greatly to the interest of an enemy to know what the psychiatrist thinks of his patient, ordinary caution would suggest that the psychiatrist speak in such a manner that it would be very difficult to put together what he says into any very definite reflection of his opinion.

This is a matter of the confidential relation of the expert and his client, which is deeply ingrained in our culture, and which we can't easily suspend. If we do choose to suspend it for cause, then I trust we will be very skillful indeed in avoiding the evil consequences which may flow from carrying out a role contrary to the expectations defined by the culture. A person who consults anyone with the idea of establishing a frank relationship with him has already overcome some pretty heavy inhibitions laid down by the culture. If the interviewer then chooses to violate the confidential relation, he must be very skillful in doing it, and quite sure that he has adequate cause for so doing—and I would define "adequate cause" as something closely related to movements designed to further the patient's progress toward finding more satisfactory ways of living.

Throughout the inception of the interview, the psychiatrist certainly, and any interviewer in some measure, should "know how he acts"—that is, he should have learned from experience the *usual* impression obtained of him in the particular circumstances of encountering the sort of stranger that the interviewee at first glance *seems* to be. In other words, the psychiatrist should have some idea of how he affects the stranger and how he facilitates or retards certain things that the stranger may have thought of doing. The psychiatrist should also have learned what sorts of immediate impressions he himself obtains from the appearance and initial movements and vocal behavior of another, noting that in such a relationship what one hears first from the other person, no matter how free and easy, or how conventional, represents that person's repertoire of operations to be addressed to a complete stranger. The psychiatrist, who is, in this situation, such a stranger, has the peculiar necessity of having some idea of how these operations affect him; otherwise he is as bad off as is the man on the street, who will perhaps waste hours of one's time arguing about the excellence of his first impressions.

It is useful for the therapist to review these details with great care at the start of his career, gradually catching on to what phenomena have made what impression on him; correspondingly, by observing the larger context of what the other person has done after the formal beginning of the interview, he can begin to develop dependable impressions of how he himself must have affected that person. For example, he may observe that, if a person says, "Hello, Doc," when he answers the door, he usually gives that person an impression of being very reserved and forbidding. He may, of course, find that the next person who greets him with "Hello, Doc," immediately thinks that he is a very fine fellow indeed. Nevertheless, he should note that this kind of rash friendliness—"Hello, Doc"—leads him to frown forbiddingly, which in turn leads many people to think that he is not a very pleasant person. Why should they think otherwise, when from the very first act with the psychiatrist, he registers this mood on his face? Thus it is useful to keep in mind what the *usual* reaction is, even if no one can swear that it will recur tomorrow.

If it has not occurred to the psychiatrist to sort out what his own particular classification of strangers is, and what effect these immediate impressions of his have on his own expression and other behavior—which in turn affect the interviewee's impression of him—he will not learn a great deal and will not improve very much. If he does look at his initial reactions from this really very simple sort of standpoint, then he will begin to make interesting observations. For instance, a great deal that we show on our faces does not ordinarily come into clear awareness, but "just happens," as it were, without our being "conscious" of it. Needless to say, becoming aware of such things is a particular aspect of alertness which requires some cultivation. Thus we can come to discover certain telltale things that we do "without thinking" which have a powerful effect in handicapping the favorable development of an interview situation. Then, after the general fashion of the exceedingly capable creature called man, once we have learned what the trouble is, it tends to disappear; we don't go on doing it.

To what does this "knowing," this "having learned," actually refer? Does it, for instance, mean that a really skillful psychiatrist "knows just what role to take," "just how to behave," in order to impress the patient in the way that the patient should be impressed? Yes; *but with very great qualifications.* It is much more accurate to say that the experience of the psychiatrist is synthesized into *an aptitude to do nothing exterior to his awareness* which will greatly handicap the development of the interview situation, or which will direct its development in an unnecessarily obscure way.

For example, many inexperienced interviewers, quite exterior to their awareness, communicate to their interviewees a distaste for certain types of data; and their records of interviews are conspicuous for the fact that the people they see don't seem to have lived in the particular areas contaminated by that distaste. Until such interviewers realize that they are rather unwittingly prohibiting, or forbidding, or shooing the interviewee away from a particular type of data, they continue not to encounter it. Thus, "learning how to act" is largely a matter of being aware of what one does, and aware of it in terms of how it affects the setting of the interview. As an interviewer does this, he stops doing those things which interfere with the fuller development of the interview.

As another aspect of "learning how to act"—or perhaps as a special instance of this awareness of one's actions which I have been discussing—the interviewer should learn to avoid any deliberate attempts to give an impression which it is *impossible* or *impracticably difficult* to sustain under the circumstances. A remarkable number of actions by psychiatrists to impress the patient have come to my attention. Not infrequently the impression that was to be conveyed to the client by certain more or less elaborate and studied behavior was quite out of keeping with the picture of the psychiatrist as seen by others. Thus all that could possibly come from this pomp and circumstance was a distinct feeling of puzzlement on the part of the interviewee. I doubt that an initial feeling of being puzzled by one's expert is an indication of his skill, and I scarcely need stress the inadvisability of acts which are calculated to produce impossibly good impressions, for these come too close to home in all of us.

While I have suggested that the psychiatrist must be alert to learn, insofar as possible, the immediate impression of him which is created in a stranger, I should at the same time emphasize that this is something which he cannot *know*. He can at best have a useful surmise of *alternative probabilities*, based on experience with other clients, and including the information he has picked up in the initial observation of the behavior demonstrated by this particular client. Now, why do I say surmises of at least *two* probabilities? I don't mind if the interviewer has a dozen, although it is very difficult to keep track of that many probabilities. But if he doesn't have more than one, he is operating on faith, which is the method of performance characteristic of people who never pause to doubt their heaven-sent ability to know all about another person by talking with him for five minutes. For such people, their *one* surmise of probability amounts to a certainty. But if the interviewer has *alternative* probabilities in mind, he is moved to explore further, whereupon the probability of one increases and that of the other diminishes; and by this simple device he moves toward reasonable accuracy. The best that a psychiatrist can have in the very early phases of his contact with a stranger is a surmise of perhaps two possible impressions that he may have created with that stranger. Such a conjecture is useful; it is the beginning of coming to know, rather roughly, how he impresses such people. The only way that he ever learns such things is by being careful to avoid closing his mind the moment he has a hunch.

Closing his mind prematurely is likely to be very gratifying or very distressing, depending upon his needs at the moment, but it will have very little effect in helping him to do better in later interviews.

An aphorism credited to ex-President Mary E. Woolley of Mount Holyoke comes to my mind as being well worth attention at this point. On one occasion this great lady said this, the truth of which rendered me all but speechless for hours after I first heard it: "It is often very important to distinguish between the merely very difficult and the actually impossible." The recognition that some things are impossible, and not just difficult, is a great economizer in any field involving very complex operations—and the psychiatric interview is probably a very complex operation. It is therefore useful, very early in one's contact with strangers, to have a lively realization that there are a great many things which would be wonderful if they were possible, but which, since they are *not* possible, it is well not to spend time on. For example, if you recall your personal observations in meeting people, you will realize that there are limits to how much it is possible to accomplish in the formal reception of a stranger. You may go to the door and call him in, or look up and say, "Oh, you are Mr. Jones," and follow this by getting the newcomer seated and so on. Such simple and conventional operations are about all that is possible at this stage with any conceivably understood result—and everything in the psychiatric interview should be sharply focused on *quite easily understood results.* When I say "understood," I refer to data that fairly readily fall into alternative hypotheses as to their probable meaning, which alternative hypotheses can then be tracked down, so that one hypothesis gains in meaning and the other fades into unimportance.

I would now like to sum up much of what I have been saying, in another aphorism which may be credited to me: *The interviewer should be alert to, so that he can correctly recall, all that he has said and done in the formal inception of each interview, so that he can learn to do better.* It is only when an interviewer can recall a course of events correctly, both as to movement and pattern of movement—that is, the timing of movement, what preceded what, what followed what—that he has the material from which to make a useful analysis of the processes which were involved, from which, in turn, he can synthesize an improving grasp of the particular aspect of living concerned. Since the interviewer is trying to be an expert at assessing the movements of another so as to get a useful view of this other person, his training may well start with the idea that he must be intensely alert to just what he himself says and does. Sometimes a patient mentions some incredible error which the psychiatrist made long past. If the psychiatrist has a vivid recall of what he said or did, the discovery that this was an incredible error might be a big step forward. Very often, however, the psychiatrist does not have any precise idea of what he did. The patient tells him something that sounds very much like what he vaguely recalls, but he doesn't know the facts clearly enough to be sure, for he was not alert enough at the time. He only knows that some serious misinterpretation has occurred of something which went on between him and the patient, which is regrettable; but so far as I know, regrets don't do people much good.

Thus one learns to devote an immense amount of alertness to the work at hand—a sort of watchful clarity as to what happens. That doesn't mean that the interviewer acts as if he were afraid that the stranger will blow up in his face, or anything like that. People can be so alert as to have a microscopically correct record of small events and yet engage congenially in all sorts of things that don't require any particular attention. And the interviewer learns that there is communication from the first visual encounter with the stranger—not only communication by speech, but communication by gesture, broadly conceived, an interchange by expressive movement other than speech.[1] That which is communicated starts the growth by inference of working hypotheses about the other person.

[1] A notion of the extent of this interchange can be obtained from the "Tentative Classification of Expressive Movements," pp. 24–35, in Gordon W. Allport and Philip E. Vernon, *Studies in Expressive Movement;* New York, Macmillan, 1933.

The Reconnaissance

As I have already suggested, by the end of the first stage the patient should have come to feel, "Well, now the doctor knows why I'm here." The psychiatrist can then say, in effect, "Well, who are you?" In other words, he sets out in this second stage to obtain a rough social sketch of the patient, which is to be brief, and not an extended life history. This is the stage to which I refer as the reconnaissance.

I customarily begin this stage by saying, "Now, tell me, how old are you? Where were you born? Are your mother and father living?" And if one or both of them are dead, "When did they die and of what?" If the patient doesn't know what his father died of, for example, this may lead to the discovery that the father hasn't lived in the home for the past twenty years, and that while the patient is pretty sure his father is dead, he doesn't know any of the circumstances. Here are some interesting data. Next I inquire as to the number of siblings, including any who died. If a sibling died during the memory span of the patient, that may be quite significant, but it is also important to note those siblings who died before he can remember, because they might have been of particular significance to his parents and thus have a considerable effect on him. I ask about his place in the time-order of siblings, and I try to get it right. Then I ask who, besides the parents, was chronically or frequently in the home in his first seven years. For example, if grandma—or a maiden aunt, or even the sheriff—was very frequently in the home during those years, this may leave a quite permanent effect; it is wise to be warned as early as possible of this, because otherwise one may make great mistakes in induction. Sorting out such data is truly impressive to a great many people. They may have actually forgotten that grandma was the one bright spot in the home in their first seven years, and are glad to be reminded of it.

I then ask what the father, or the mother, or whoever earned the money, did for a living. I probably by now have derived a notion of the family's economic circumstances—if I haven't,

I ask specifically. I then ask if there was any sharp change in the economic circumstances at any time. (All this was, of course, impressed on me because I went into private practice just as the Great Depression arrived.) Marked economic disturbances usually have either general or special reasons, and have very marked effects on the course of personality development. Parents almost always aim their children at something, which the children either seek or avoid at all costs, but big economic change may lead to tragic revision of the parental ambitions with corresponding effects on the children's goals and so on, and may leave permanent marks. If there were changes, I try to notice how old the patient was when they occurred. If they occurred very early, before the patient was eight, they may have greatly influenced the parental utterances and efforts to direct the life of the child. If the changes occurred when the patient was around twenty, they may have affected his getting a university education—or if he was headed for medicine or the law, they may have affected his educational goal even though he was older. If the changes occurred after he completed his education, they have probably not made very much difference except insofar as they have made other people dependent on him.

And when I have all this information—and note that I am proceeding in what has gradually been ingrained in me as a system of values that seems natural to Americans—I become curious, sometimes to the patient's amazement, as to what sort of a person his father was. People are anything from extremely vocal to helpless in the face of such a question, and if a patient's helplessness seems to be a real lack of verbal formulation, I say, "Well, how was he regarded in the community?" If he still cannot formulate this, I may mention the pastor of the church, and the family doctor, and the druggist with whom he had an account, and the grocer, and so on, asking, "What would they have said of him, offhand?"

A slight haste in the face of obscurity does no harm here, because brevity about these things is not solely for the physician's convenience; it also has a certain relevance in the matter of what the patient is there for. You see, he really isn't there to give me an adequate biography of himself; and so, if I seem a little hurried in getting what I want of his biography, his grievance is minimal. When I have obtained some idea of what sort of person the father was, I become curious to learn whether it was a happy family. Were the parents happily married? Then I want to know about the mother. And for reasons that I would never try to put into words, while I ask *what sort of a person* the father was, I ask the patient to *describe* his mother. When we have developed this point somewhat—the patient usually has an exceedingly vague idea of the lady—I then remember any other stray people who were mentioned earlier as being around the house a great deal in the very early years and ask what sort of people they were. This is usually such a relief to the patient after trying to describe his mother that I often get quite an account of the third, the semiparent; and that semiparent may prove to be illuminating, if only in understanding the role that I may play later on in the relationship.

At this point, I usually sigh—for sufficient reason—and ask the patient to tell me something about his education; and when we have gone through that as rapidly as possible, I want to know his occupational history. In the educational history, I don't believe I'd waste a minute with most people to find out whether or not they were held back in a grade in grammar school, unless I felt that they were probably feeble-minded. Education is, so far as I am concerned, a clear index of the combination of foresight and blind ambition on the part of parents, wealthy relatives, and the patient. The educational history can be quite, quite brief, such as, "Well, I went from high school to such-and-such a prep school, and then to such-and-such a college, and I finally got a Ph.D. from such-and-such a place." That is enough; it merely tells me that he is lucky, as the average person goes.

The occupational history, while it still includes big factors of the general economic situation, the particular geographical opportunities, and so on, is much more illuminating as to the patient's ability to get on with people and to get somewhere in life. Therefore, I now want to know what he has done ever since leaving school, and I am rather curious about this. The sicker people are, the more they omit from their occupational history. And so here, for the first time, I quite generally do something which is a very important part of the psychiatric interview: I tell the patient what I have heard, and then inquire whether that is the whole story, by saying something like, "Well, aside from these two jobs you have had no other occupation?" Whereupon many people reveal that, oh, yes, they have had twenty-five other jobs, but they haven't held them long. This is much more important information than that about the two jobs mentioned first. Thus one should discover whether or not there is more occupational history than the interviewee at first reports. However, I watch the clock as I do it. That is, I don't want to know how bad the foreman was; all I want to know is what jobs, how long, and where—thus getting an idea of whether the person was advancing in his work; whether he was so driven by a need for money that he held a job only long enough to get one that paid more; whether he held each job long enough to know what the work was about and then took another one, in a curiously thorough but superficially morbid pattern of learning something about life; whether he quarreled with everybody that he ever tried to work with; and all that sort of thing. I don't want details, but I do want a sketch of the facts.

At this point I become curious as to whether the person is married, and if so, how long he has been married. I ask somewhat casually, "Quite happily?" And if it isn't a happy marriage, the patient usually takes a moment to say "Yes." Sometimes I look at him then, and ask if there are any children; and I may ask if it is the first marriage. Quite often a person will say, "No, no, I was married before," sounding as if I should have known this, when everything he has said so far was not in any sense calculated to suggest such a thing. Then I want to know about the early marriage. The great thing is: Was it the first love?—and if there is a little hesitancy there, then comes, of course, the inquiry, "Why did you marry?" Sometimes it was just because the family thought it was a great idea. I receive all this information without surprise, for an expert is not surprised at getting what he wants.

With that I'm through. Of the labels which the patient's neighbors and casual acquaintances attach to him, I have tried to pick up those that have some measure of probable significance for understanding what he does. He feels that I know a great deal about him—in part because a good deal of these data are ordinarily not discussed in his relations with strangers. In a vague way, I do know a good deal, because from now on I just watch which of the customary indices prove to be correct in his case, and wherein he is an exception to the probabilities which are implied in the semistatistical data of his past, his family position, and so on.

For example, there is some probability that the fifth and last child in a family, who is the only male child, and who is born ten years after his nearest sibling, will be dreadfully spoiled. On discovering that a person occupies that position in the family, I immediately think, "Hah! The probability is that this fellow has gotten away with murder since his early years." And so I notice this, I begin with it, but I hope that I recognize any very striking exceptions that I encounter. That is what the brief sketch is for. The interviewer utilizes as much as he can of the dubious, but still respectable, generalizations that he has picked up in all his previous life and study, remembering, however, that those generalizations are statements of probability; they are never statements to the effect that "under these circumstances so-and-so is inevitably the case." We don't have that sort of absolute knowledge about human living, and, therefore, we shall remain eternally young. If it turns out that *nothing* about the patient fits with any of the interviewer's past experience, he will really have a grand and difficult task in being useful to this patient.

Some psychiatrists, having discovered that someone is the youngest child and the only male, born many years after the nearest sibling, consider it a certainty, rather than a probability, that he is dreadfully spoiled. Those folks ought to go into the natural sciences, rather than deal with human living. The exceptions to the probabilities which arise from this type of crude data about people are very striking. They may not approximate 50 per cent, but they are still a very significant group of exceptions; and since the interviewer is supposed to show some expertness in dealing with people, it is well for him not to close his mind to them. But insofar as the probabilities that he has come to accept hold true in a given case, those data are easy to keep track of from then on. And when he encounters exceptions, simply because everyone is respectful of exceptions from their very nature of being somewhat against the rule, he finds them a little easier to recall than if he had blundered into them somewhat blindly while listening to a long life history and perhaps getting all wrapped up in Aunt Hattie's peculiar attacks that came on at the menopause, which are relevant only if one is curious as to whether there is lunacy in the family, which can be a dreadful waste of time.

Thus the second step is a very hurried picking up of the kind of clues which ordinarily can be rather useful in considering anybody's personality and habits. But notice that I haven't asked anything about the person's personality; I have simply tried to find out how he comes to be here—in the sense of time and space—to find out what the grossest landmarks are that have characterized his course up to now. Nevertheless, by the time these gross social data have been completed, the psychiatrist will have been impressed with many characteristics of the person with whom he is dealing. Because of the great number of topics covered in the social outline, and because of their real importance and yet apparent lack of relationship, the patient is much more apt to show meaningful signs, without perhaps quite knowing it, than would be the case if he were conversing freely about something in which he more or less had control of the topics. Later on, in the detailed inquiry, unless for some reason the psychiatrist really must resort to cross-examination, it is to a large extent necessary to leave the patient more or less in control of the topics; things have to flow, for otherwise they are apt to be so disconnected that the interviewer does not quite know what he has learned.

But in the reconnaissance, in which the interviewee is more or less answering an organized stream of questions, the interviewer has an opportunity, by alert listening and some seeing, to pick up a great many clues for further exploration. For example, the interviewer notes in this stage the relative ease or difficulty of the relationship, which reflects the degree of the interviewee's concentration on the procedure; his sensitivity to the other person—in this instance, the interviewer; and his "attitudes," as one commonly describes them in such terms as reserved, guarded, suspicious, hostile, defensive, conciliatory, apologetically inferior, superior, supercilious, mutually respecting. The interviewer may also observe the interviewee's attitude toward his own memory—whether he seems to trust it or not; his attitude about "answering questions"—whether this makes him feel at a disadvantage or not; the apparent extent of his need for reassurance; and so on. Later on, when I discuss the interview as a process, I will discuss in more detail the kinds of gross impressions which the interviewer can gather during this stage of the interview, and the ways in which he evaluates these impressions and tests their validity.

The Reconnaissance in Intensive Psychotherapy [2]

The reconnaissance may take about twenty minutes, in a case where I never expect to see the person again, or it may take from seven and a half to fifteen hours, which I think is about the average when time is not of the essence, or it may take even longer. Once in my actual experience, literally a little over three months was spent in this phase which I call the reconnaissance; the person concerned was a candidate in training who had done a great deal of thinking about his personal history, and therefore the personal history itself was rather rich in data, and already pretty well organized.

The skill which an interviewer can manifest in obtaining and interpreting this outline history has a great deal to do with

[2] [Editors' note: The remainder of this chapter is taken from a series of lectures on *Conceptions of Modern Psychiatry*, which Sullivan gave in the Washington School of Psychiatry in 1946-47, and in which he discussed some aspects of psychiatric interviewing.]

the ease or difficulty of the subsequent detailed inquiry—
which, if the interviewer is a psychiatrist undertaking treatment of a patient, ordinarily means the long stretch of intensive
psychotherapy. Depending on the concise accuracy of the
outstanding points in this reconnaissance sketch of the personality, the detailed inquiry may be reduced, I suppose, as much
as 90 per cent.[3] I am quite sure that the reason for the unending
spans of lifetime spent in supposed intensive psychotherapy of
patients is in some instances simply the fact that the psychiatrist
had no particular hints of how the particular patient had got
to be the person who had come to the office; instead, the psychiatrist depended on what is called free association to find all
that out. Since association can be extremely free indeed, by the
time that the psychiatrist had some notion of the life history
of the patient I'm afraid he had the wrong notion. Thus the
ideal time to make this sort of inquiry—to try to find out "How
come this patient?" in terms of his rudimentary life history—
is right after the thing has begun, as soon as a potential doctor-
patient relationship has been established. If the doctor does
that, then he is in a position to have views which are not

[3] [*Editors' note:* In a question-and-answer session at the end of the 1944
series of lectures, Sullivan made the following remarks in response to a question about brief psychotherapy:

"I have long held that 'brief' psychotherapy was to be achieved by improving the utilization of the psychotherapeutic minute. If one is governed
by no principles, but only by some vague beliefs—as in something like 'free
association'—I think brief psychotherapy is very likely to be measured in
terms of decades. But if one is interested in a precisely defined, recurrent
difficulty that people have in significant relations to others, it is quite possible
that a good deal can be done in a rather short time. If a good deal *is* to be
done in a short time, neither the patient nor the doctor can permit long
sustained digressions about their mutual admirability, or about interesting
shows in the theater, or something of the sort. In fact, the psychiatrist must
follow events closely enough so that whenever a digression seems to be in
progress, or some subordinate problem seems to be in the center of things,
he can inquire whether such is truly the case, or whether the topic actually
does fit in with the business before them. In those circumstances, the patient
may come to see that the psychiatrist knows what he is doing, and that there
is good reason to collaborate in doing it. Incidentally, I think that the frequency of interview is important only from the standpoint of the limitations
of the psychiatrist; and that is a matter of his ability to recall. It usually takes
me a little while, in each interview, to recall what has been going on; usually
the patient says something which brings up the right recognition, and we
are then off to where we were at the time of the previous session."]

transcendental. And even if half the facts told him then are wrong, they will be corrected fairly soon.

Suppose, on the other hand, that a person comes to the psychiatrist and says, "I've been diagnosed as an obsessional neurotic and told I need psychoanalysis. Can you take me?" and the psychiatrist says, "Yes, let us begin." What is assumed there? First, that a competent diagnosis has been made; and second, that the psychiatrist is a godlike person who is bound to be successful—or that he is an unprincipled scoundrel who will take money without any thought of what the patient is going to get for it. I suggest that a psychiatrist find out something about a person before he makes or implies expansive promises about what he will do, or what ought to be done, and particularly before he begins to do something which may or may not have any earthly constructive influence on the patient. I insist that the psychiatrist should in the beginning try to find out something about the patient, not in the sense of developing a psychiatric history according to this or that outline which he may find in the mental hospital library, but from the standpoint of orienting himself as to certain basic probabilities according to the developmental scheme of things.

I do not mean to imply that all of the reconnaissance is always rather sharply separated from all of the detailed inquiry. In actual fact, there are matters that come up in such a way in the course of developing this social outline that it is obviously highly advantageous to pursue the topic immediately in detail. It is very much better to go into the details when it is opportune than to be in any sense obsessional about following the rest of the social outline before getting anything to hang on it. Unless something is deferred smoothly and in a fashion which the interviewee experiences as natural, it is not apt to be the same thing when it comes up again. For example, in inquiring about the mother, the interviewer may have learned that she was a wonderful woman, except that she had a violent temper and at times really seemed a little bit out of her mind from anger. If, after he has heard a statement like that, he then shifts to an inquiry about someone else, the patient is apt to suffer over the baldness of his original statement. As a result, when the interviewer gets around to asking about the mother again, he may hear a stream of apologies about what was first said, the patient having by then convinced himself that it is necessary to be much less frank in his statements. By this time the interviewer cannot be nearly so sure of what he is getting. But if, when the original statement is made, the interviewer invites a few examples—what sort of thing was apt to precipitate the mother's violent anger, and so on—before going on with other matters, then the topic is opened wide, and eventually the details may be gone into with much less distress.

THE USE OF FREE ASSOCIATION

During the reconnaissance, the interviewer may hear of some situation at some time in the patient's past which seems significant, but which is unclear; when the interviewer asks supplementary questions, he may get to a point where something he would like to know is not accessible to the patient. The patient is unable to recall it; to use the old slang, the material has been "repressed." Here is an opportunity to do something very educative. The interviewer may say, "Well, I really wonder what might have been the case; tell me, what comes to your mind?" Partly because of the pressure, partly because of the objectivity of the inquiry, and partly because the patient really is trying to get something out of his contact with psychiatry, he often has a very surprising experience indeed in discovering what comes to his mind. In other words, by attacking blind spots in the patient's recollection in this very simple way, the interviewer is actually giving him a hint as to the nature of free association that might be terribly hard to give otherwise.

As a matter of fact, trying to tell patients what is meant by free association, and trying to get them to do it, can be quite a problem. I used to collect prescriptions given to patients by analysts about how to go to work. Of course, the first instruction in the old days was, "Lie down on the couch and relax completely." One of unnumbered variants of this prescription went on, "Feel as much at peace as possible, and say every littlest thing that comes to your mind." Trying to relax completely always stymied the patient, so the psychiatrist didn't have to worry about anything else for a while; some patients could spend the next six months trying to relax completely, without one success. If the psychiatrist tells patients to do things that they can't do, they very rarely have the good sense to say, "Yes, Doctor, how do you do it?" Instead, they just presume that the psychiatrist knows what he's talking about, and try. If the prescription doesn't work, such patients then have proof that they can't get any benefit from psychiatry.

None of these prescriptions ever got anywhere in my hands. I finally concluded that the only way to get a patient to doing free association that is of any good to him or to me is to impress upon him the faculty of his personality to present unknown data by more or less free flow of thought. And I also concluded that the way to impress this on him was not by talking about it, but by having a few demonstrations of it. The ideal circumstance for this is when a valid question arises and the patient has nothing in the way of an answer. Thus, when we take up some problem that has emerged in the reconnaissance, and run into blind areas concerning it—that is, areas where the self-system is at work—I try to get the patient to talk more or less at random as things come to his mind; and then, as often as not, the patient gives a very convincing demonstration of moving toward useful information. In other words, when the patient has no answer for a question which is obviously of real importance to him, the functioning of the personality is such that the following process is likely to ensue: as the patient begins to talk about the things that come to his mind, his thoughts will begin to circle, in the most curious fashion, toward the answering of the question. It may be, of course, that the process will start and stop many a time before a very significant question is answered.

Only after the patient has had a few examples of the fact that free association makes sense can the psychiatrist lay down injunctions about it—even useful injunctions as to the inadvisability of his selecting what to report. When the patient has actually accomplished something by a more or less free report of his covert processes, he will begin to understand that the leaving out of ideas because they seem irrelevant or immaterial may cause the therapeutic process to miscarry. I have often heard people start out on what seemed to be a simple evasion of an anxiety-fraught position—that is, they seemed to be talking about something irrelevant; but if they were really faithfully reporting what went on in their minds, it wasn't irrelevant very long, for the mind usually does not spend much time on irrelevant and unimportant details. Of course, when a person keeps on talking about the bees and the flowers, and so on, I may say quite sardonically, "This seems to be *really* free association, but I wonder what on earth it pertains to."

Thus my way of getting this very valuable aspect of personality to work is to induct the patient into the reporting of relatively free-flowing thought before giving him any hint that that is a very important method. One might think that everybody by now knows all about free association, and cannot be entrapped into doing it by such a simple technique. But if you are doing a fairly good job of the reconnaissance, patients are much too interested and busy to be thinking about the latest psychoanalytic movie they have seen, for they are really at work on something of importance to them. So the psychiatrist should try to get something to *happen*, that he can then refer to as having happened, instead of telling the patient to say every littlest thing that comes to his mind, or something of the sort.

SUMMARIZING THE RECONNAISSANCE

In my proxy [4] experience of the last three years, I have found it useful to recommend that the psychiatrist—particularly in a series of interviews with one patient—conclude the preliminary reconnaissance with a summary statement. Thus the summary statement would be made at the end of, say, seven to fifteen hours of interviews, and it would precede the detailed

[4] [*Editors' note:* Sullivan is referring here to his supervisory and consultative work with psychotherapists in the Washington area.]

efforts of psychotherapy. In this summary statement, the psychiatrist tells the patient what he has heard and what he sees as a problem that seems well within the field of psychiatric competence. In my experience, such a statement has without exception proved extremely useful to the patient and gratifying to the therapist. In fact, even in cases where a patient who was being seen for a single interview was enraged by the summary, and apparently closed the door to all psychiatric help, I have sometimes found out later through collateral information that the patient was benefited. In a long series of interviews, it is important to establish the justifiability of the patient's seeing the psychiatrist; the relationship should not be left tacit as to its basic nature for very long. The psychiatric situation is formally established when there is a consensus—even if unwilling—that the patient and the psychiatrist might well talk further about the problem which has emerged from the reconnaissance.

The summary at the end of the reconnaissance should be presented with as much economy of time as possible, short of rudeness; if the psychiatrist is prolix at this time the patient is likely to become vastly more prolix in the course of the detailed inquiry. In presenting the summary, the psychiatrist should explain that he now wishes to tell the patient what has impressed him in the reconnaissance, and that he would like the patient to bear with him until he is through, so that he will be relatively uninterrupted; at the same time, the psychiatrist should tell the patient that at the end of the summary the patient will be asked to amend and correct those things which the psychiatrist has misunderstood, and to point out any important things which the psychiatrist has missed.

Many therapists on first attempting to use this method have encountered remarkable impulses in themselves to procrastinate about summarizing, and have felt profoundly uncertain as to what to put in the summary, and so on; in fact, they usually have had to make an extraordinarily firm resolve before actually getting around to summarizing. I have great sympathy with the psychiatrist's reluctance to tell the patient what he

has learned about him. As psychiatrists, we can all advance the
perfectly reasonable argument that psychiatry is a very complex field and that, at a given time in therapy with a patient, we
haven't had enough time to verify the facts. Many psychiatrists
who have not had the experience of using the summary statement have a gloomy feeling which might be verbalized somewhat as follows: "If I were to tell the patient how little I've
caught on to of what he has told me, he'd be completely discouraged." But the brute fact is that in all of my experience by
proxy with this procedure, this gloomy anticipation of how
badly the psychiatrist will show himself up with the patient
has never been realized once; in each instance, the summary
has resulted in the patient's showing a very marked respect for
the psychiatrist. The psychiatrist, you see, is peculiarly quali-
fied—by virtue of his psychiatric education—to sort out the
relevant details of another person's life and throw them into
meaningful patterns, as compared with any of the infinite
number of voluntary advisers that the patient, like everybody
else, has been dealing with previously.

One of the reasons for the psychiatrist's initial hesitancy in
revealing by means of a summary how at sea he feels in the
interview situation is that the sort of things that he summarizes
is determined by his own experience and his own grasp on
living. That is what is behind the feeling of helplessness that we
all have at times in undertaking a summary. But the psychiatrist's own limitations of experience and lack of grasp on living
are handicaps in working with the patient, particularly in the
detailed inquiry, whether or not the psychiatrist is aware of
them. In addition, sometimes it is actually beneficial for the
patient to realize that the psychiatrist, because of his own experience, is somewhat insensitive to certain areas of living. The
most crushing outcome of such a revelation would be that the
patient would find another psychiatrist, which in some cases
might be of real usefulness for the first psychiatrist if he were
able to learn something from it.

When the psychiatrist seriously attempts to summarize what
has happened at the end of the reconnaissance, the patient will

have an experience which in some ways is quite startling. Things that the patient has known all of his life and which he has told the psychiatrist in the interviews will be reflected back to him in the summary in a newly meaningful fashion—in spite of what the psychiatrist thinks of as his own stupidities and forgetfulnesses. Thus to the extent that the summary represents a somewhat expert view of the data that the patient had accessible in his awareness and was moved to report in the interview, it will be a very uplifting experience to the patient —a very definite step in the patient's education as to how psychiatry works. And quite often the summary shows the patient some of his conventional evasions and distortions.

In presenting the summary, the psychiatrist has to use some judgment in determining when he has an outline of reasonably significant things; and he will never know how good his judgment is in that respect until he has tried it. After the psychiatrist has summarized the situation and given a sort of recommendation of what he feels might well be more or less the point of immediate attack, he should, as I have said, encourage the patient to amend and correct the statement. Real amendment and correction on the part of the patient are important, for, in this way, the psychiatrist can learn a lot more about what he has on his hands than he could find out in the same time by any other means. In fact, this is an immensely good way of getting things started on something like a consensually valid basis. Of course, if the psychiatrist sees that the patient is merely amending in an obsessional way—just gilding the lily— he should interrupt the patient and say, "Yes, yes. Well, I gather that you're in approximate agreement with my view. Of course, I can't cover all the details that you've covered."

Actually most of the patient's amending at the end of the summary has consisted, in my own experience, of reminding me that I have dropped out some important figure. In those cases in which two or three people had much the same influence on the patient's difficulties in living, I quite often forget all but one of these people. And the patient at the end will think, "But where was Aunt Agatha?" and mention the fact that I have forgotten the importance of this figure. He is unable at that juncture to generalize about these figures; but he is quite content when I say, "Oh, yes, Aunt Agatha was also like such-and-such a person." He then sees that I am aware of the important experience, even if I don't recall all the significant figures. In the single interview of an hour and a half, I have often used a ten-minute summary at the end of an hour and fifteen minutes to try to tell the patient what I thought was quite important in what I had heard. The patient may sputter around for the last five minutes about what I have left out of the summary, but quite often he ends the interview by indicating that he will follow my suggestion about what to do next, in this way indicating that my summary has been of use to him. Despite the fact that the psychiatrist will leave many gaps in this brief summary, he should be able to give the patient a clear notion of what he considers an important problem.

Somewhat tangentially, I would like to mention that it is useful in a series of interviews to have the patient prepare a chronology of his life. This is quite helpful for a psychiatrist like myself who has great difficulty in getting abstract names attached to concrete people. In addition, it saves time in dealing with patients who are particularly productive of names and who mention, in the course of the work, everybody with whom they have had any dealings. I suggest that the patient prepare a record, showing in one column the date or the year and his age, beginning with his birth and coming up to the present, and in another column, opposite this time scale, brief statements of where he lived, who was living in the household at the given time, and any very significant events, including those that he has been telling me about. I explain that such a record might help him to recall certain things that had not shown up in the early reconnaissance and that it would be very valuable to me in keeping track of the various people and when their influence was felt by the patient. I point out that this will save a good deal of time for both of us, and that it will help me to avoid misunderstandings. Very frequently, indeed, the patient adopts this suggestion and both of us profit from this procedure.

The question of what to include in the summary, in terms of the patient's problem as the psychiatrist sees it, is a very real one. To be simply frank in psychiatric work would often result in a situation in which the psychiatrist was as cruel and destructive as possible. When we later consider the development of the self-system, it will become somewhat clearer that a great many people are easily exposed to extremely severe anxiety unless they can maintain certain conventional defensive operations which represent the anti-anxiety manifestations of the self. The psychiatrist therefore always has the responsibility of presenting a problem in the patient's living in such a way that it does something more than precipitate intense anxiety. At the end of the reconnaissance it is possible for the psychiatrist to present problems in such a way that the patient won't become too anxious to continue to work with that psychiatrist. In some instances, I have given a patient a rather grim statement at the end of, say, seven hours that would have terminated treatment had I tossed it out as a conclusion at the end of the first hour. But in the period of the reconnaissance the patient has had hints that the encounter makes sense and that the psychiatrist did not put things as brutally, unfeelingly, contemptuously, and superiorly as possible; and these earlier hints have made it possible for the patient to rally from the effect of the rather grim summary.

Perhaps an example might illustrate the sort of summary that can be useful without being too anxiety-provoking. In commenting on a patient's particular pattern of disparagement of others, I might say, "Well, it seems to me that this pattern of giving lip service and then undermining the other person, which you were forced to develop with Aunt Agatha, has stayed with you ever since." If said in another way, this might be extremely offensive to the patient and intensely provocative of insecurity. But such a pattern of behavior, when placed in its historic setting, does not seem quite as horrible as when it is placed in a more immediate context. Once the patient is able to recall what I'm talking about in that setting, then I can say, "Well, this pattern seems to have gone on, huh?" In a vague way, there's a sort of transfer of blame to Aunt Agatha in this approach. More important, I have indicated that I am interested in how things began, and that I am not surprised that some of them go on still, even though the patient has not recognized this pattern up to now and, having recognized it, is not particularly happy about it.

Sometimes the problems in living which the psychiatrist encounters in the reconnaissance are so grave, so close to the structure of the most serious mental disorders, that it would be simply disastrous to toss them in the patient's face. The psychiatrist cannot expect a patient who is deeply disturbed to give up his shadowy vestiges of security by agreeing with the psychiatrist that he is psychotic. Even in those cases, however, I believe that the patient should be presented with something. If the psychiatrist omits all emphasis on what in the patient's behavior actually demonstrates psychosis, he can sometimes refer to what are in essence the patient's psychotic difficulties with others, without actually communicating the idea to the patient that these difficulties constitute a particular very severe mental disorder. Under those circumstances, it is by no means uncommon for the patient to be quite clear on the fact that in a rather objective and undisturbing fashion, the psychiatrist has said, in essence, that he is psychotic; and this is established without any serious movement of anxiety, and with the patient's feeling that it might be possible to get somewhere with the psychiatrist.

Perhaps a case which I happen to remember at the moment will illustrate some of the points that I have been making about the summary. Some time ago, I had occasion to see a patient who revealed in the first interview that he had a homosexual problem. The upshot of the reconnaissance was that I told him that I had no psychiatric time available—and I didn't know anybody else who had—for his interest in homosexual problems. If, on the other hand, he wanted to find out why he could never hold any one job for more than six months—despite an initial curiously ascending progress at amazing speed—and was always in ever-increasing, terrific danger of being completely discredited and expelled by the organization he worked for, then I thought I could find him a psychiatrist. Believe it or not, the patient was quite content to go to work on the problem of why, in the space of six months or so, each one of his bosses came into such open collision with him that he left. The curious thing about this story is that in the process of studying his difficulties with bosses, the great homosexual problem sort of caved in. This kind of success story doesn't happen very often; in general, homosexual problems or any other problems don't just cave in. The important part of this story is that, as a result of a brief reconnaissance, I declined entirely to have anything to do with what the patient considered his problem. Instead I indicated a problem that needed very urgent treatment and that I thought psychiatry could help him with. The patient agreed, and we went to work on this second problem—that is, we began the detailed inquiry.

Thus in my summary of the reconnaissance, I strive always to outline for a patient what I see as a major difficulty of his living which seems well within the field of psychiatry. In doing this I imply that if we work together I hope that we can get somewhere on this problem. Although I call this a major problem, I have no prestige whatever involved in its being *the* major problem of the patient's life, or the one that we will spend many months on in a long series of interviews. As a matter of fact, many people cannot bring into the open the major problem of their living until they have found themselves in an almost impossibly secure interpersonal situation. In such cases, it may well be long after the reconnaissance that *the* great major problem of living will become clear.

If by the end of the reconnaissance, the interviewer is not able to clearly define any major problem of the patient, he should not be at all hesitant to indicate something quite minor that ails the patient. Perhaps the patient may think, "Oh, yes, but that's just a trifle; the doctor just doesn't know what really ails me." But the patient also knows that the reason the doctor is unclear about the more important problems is that the patient couldn't show them to the doctor. And if the doctor has stated a problem, however minor, in an adequate fashion, this statement has not foreclosed all sorts of discoveries in the future; he has merely indicated that, so far as he is concerned, this problem is worth working on. The important thing is that the doctor and patient now have something to work on.

Without this statement of a problem in living, treatment situations are apt to be quite defeating. They are painfully reminiscent of the steel plant where I once worked; after a sleet storm, the little narrow-gauge locomotives with their loads of ingots would struggle along the icy tracks and progress would apparently be made, when suddenly everything would slide back to just where it had been before. In the psychiatric interview, this business of much ado, no achievement, and a sort of aching void, in which the doctor must try to whip up excitement again, can all be remedied by the simple expedient of establishing something to work on at the end of the reconnaissance. The doctor then goes to work on that particular problem. If the patient seems to drift away from that problem to no purpose, the doctor investigates what has happened. But if the patient moves from this problem to something which seems to be much more important, then the doctor can rest. The point is that the psychiatrist tries to have something to work on, and he continues to work on it until something more worthy of his attention comes along. And in some ways that's the whole story of intensive psychotherapy.

CHAPTER
V

The Detailed Inquiry: The Theoretical Setting

DURING THE early stages of the interview, the interviewer will have received a good many impressions of the sort of person whom he is participantly observing. These impressions derived from the two initial phases of an interview should stand him in very good stead in quickly putting into effect the procedures which make up the long haul of actual detailed inquiry. Most unhappily, these impressions will be in need of a great deal of revision as a series of interviews proceed, or even during one long interview. Again I say that impressions are, in their purer sense, hypotheses, and like every other hypothesis they should be tested. Thus the impressions that one gains during the first two stages are tested in the prolonged detailed inquiry.

From my years of experience with the interview I would say that there are enough merits in one's early impressions of a stranger to justify some conceit. But this fact can become a very great handicap to any distinguished success in interviewing, since there are enough instances of singularly incorrect impressions to justify a very thorough realization that one must constantly test alternatives and try to keep an open mind as to the essential correctness of his impressions. It is foolish to assume that one's first impression is any good except in a very general sense. There is no magic by which even the most experienced human being can assess in a relatively simple series of relationships the dependable patterns of another personality.

Nor can the psychiatrist determine after a few interviews the durable characteristics of a patient so accurately that predictions can be made of the patient's performance in any given situation. I know no evidence whatsoever that any such magic can be performed. If the interviewer finds that his impressions at the start of an interview situation have been rather close to his impressions at the end of an interview, then he can feel immensely encouraged; it is another of the unnumbered manifestations of the extraordinarily gifted character of the human being. But if the interviewer begins to rest on his laurels by assuming that an early impression of a stranger has more than purely experimental importance, then he is not yet ready to do interviewing.

The stage of detailed inquiry in the psychiatric interview is a matter of improving on earlier approximations of understanding, in which process a really revolutionary change in one's impressions may occur. A good many times I have had to make really phenomenal revisions of early impressions of a patient, on the basis of data in the detailed inquiry. Often the statements that misled me would have misled anyone who was paying attention only to what these statements *presumably* meant. For example, patients may tell a psychiatrist things which have so little to do with their durable characteristics that he finally realizes that one of the great difficulties in the interview is the patient's effort to suit him, to impress him. Although this is not a matter of deliberate malice or of stupidity on the patient's part, it does subtly color the way things are presented. Thus the patient is completely unaware of any intention of deceiving the psychiatrist or defeating him in his efforts to find out what is going on; and things which are actually grossly misleading get themselves said as simply as if they were absolute truths.

This element of unreliability in making responses to questions is not uniquely a part of the psychiatric interview. In any life situation, when a person is asked a question his reply varies greatly in its appropriateness, significance, communicativeness, and so on, according to what area of contact with reality the question seems to pertain to. I can ask you, for example, how to get from your house to the nearest streetcar stop, with a high probability that I will get a communicative response. Questions of geometric or geographical orientation addressed to a hundred persons in series would bring something like forty responses which would be incomplete and very much off the point. However, more than fifteen out of a hundred answers would be responsive to the question, and prove to be fairly adequate reflections of what might be described as fixed aspects of reality.

In this realm of alleged spatial relationships which have no particular significance except their immediate utility to the person involved, one can expect some degree of adequacy in the response. In the next category of relationships—those which refer to time—there seems to be an increase in the fringe of irrelevance, uncertainty, misinformation, and so on. If I were to ask a group of sightseers, "Did you go to this place or that place first?" I would discover from the answers that there is not nearly as high a probability that the honest, solemnly helpful answer has any useful relationship to the facts, as those facts would be perceived by a third person, or revealed in a crude statistical analysis of the actual data.

We could proceed to study, through gradation after gradation, the probability of a particular request for information calling out something usefully related to a significant course of events. When in this long series of gradations, which I shall not attempt to outline now, we would finally come to questions about one's belief about how one should act under a given situation—such as asking several people, "How do you believe that you *should* behave about so and so?"—amazingly enough we would find that the responses contained practically no uncertainty; suddenly each answer would be very close to the so-called norm of conduct in that particular. Now if we were to alter the question a little and ask, "How *did* you act under such-and-such circumstances?" referring now to a real event, the answers would be really amazing; the fringe of irrelevancy in the replies, the immateriality of them, and so on, would closely approximate 100 per cent. In other words, a person can't tell you accurately how he acted in an important situation unless by almost sheer chance the way he *did* act happened to coincide with his idea of how he *should* have acted—a rather uncommon coincidence in which the answer is just as good as a geographical direction. In other words, everyone knows in a particular cultural situation just how he ought to act. If his behavior coincides with what he thinks he ought to have done, he can report the matter accurately. If, as is very much more frequently the case, there is no such coincidence between the act and the ideal, one finds that there is a truly astonishing decrease in the likelihood of the response being valid.

Thus it seems to be almost impossible for any of us, in dealing with strangers at least, to say anything which will perfectly succinctly demonstrate that we are inferior to our demands on our own behavior. We all know when we are "at fault" about what we did—an idea which is first learned in childhood from the authority figures. When we start to report something that doesn't come up to our standard of behavior, we know that it doesn't come up to this standard. That goes on in covert processes very quickly. What we then produce, however, is no simple statement. It is a stream of words aimed at what we trust is the unskeptical ear that is listening.

The work of an interviewer is largely concerned with evaluating such statements—apologies for failure, extravagant exaggeration of successes, and studious minimization of errors. Thus the detailed part of the psychiatric interview, in order to be significant, has to be exceedingly far from a conversation made up of simple, correct answers to clear questions. The uncertainties of this part of the interview arise from the interviewee's feeling that what occurs to him isn't "good enough." The real facts of the interview situation might be expressed: "If I tell the doctor the truth, he won't think well of me." Or, "Well, I must put a good face on that; otherwise I might make a bad impression." Or again, "My God! If I do things like that, of course he won't authorize my employment." All of these covert operations show an attempt on the part of the interviewee to read the interviewer's mind. A great many of them form defects in the process of communication, for all of them spring from a dreadfully troublesome and significant question in the mind of the interviewee: "What will he think?" The complex products which the interviewer gets from the interviewee arise from the latter's attempt to avoid even the faintest sign of an unfavorable answer to that question in his mind. There isn't the remotest chance that any person in this social order, and probably in any other extant in the world today, will not try to put his best foot forward, which means that each of us in talking about any of our past performances will try to guess what we can say that will minimize the unfavorable aspects of such performances. This is such a universal phenomenon that it would be utterly absurd for an interviewer to be annoyed by all the complex answers—this walking around the obvious—that he gets from questions which he poses to the interviewee.

If we translate this phenomenon into the psychiatric situation, we find that from the psychiatrist's standpoint all of his contacts with any patient are marked by *the patient's strange dependence for some kind of comfort on what the patient believes the psychiatrist thinks of what is being discussed.* It is hardly necessary to say that the patient's idea of what the therapist is thinking about the patient's remarks is often far from accurate. When it occurs to a patient that he does not have a fair idea as to what the therapist is thinking, his distress is often pathetic. The hesitancy—the attempt to cover two horns of a dilemma with one foot—is poignant, and is really distressing to the patient. It may be much more comfortable for the patient to hold the opinion that he "knows" what the psychiatrist is driving at, that he has some idea of what the "right" answer is, and that he can with some accuracy estimate how his prestige stands with the psychiatrist, than it is to have any reasonable appreciation of the simple fact that the psychiatrist is giving forth with no signs whatsoever on which to base any reliable interpretation of the psychiatrist's attitude. When the conservation of time is quite important, it is very convenient for the psychiatrist to develop a way of behavior that gives no clear index as to his favorable or unfavorable response to what he has heard. Under those circumstances the patient usually operates under the assumption that he can accurately guess whether he is making a good impression on the psychiatrist and will get somewhere, or whether he is making a bad impression and won't. The patient feels much more comfortable if he is completely deluded in his impressions of the psychiatrist's impressions, whether or not he is working on an important aspect of his personality. Although all this seems to be an impractical way to handle the business of living, it is, I assure you, quite understandable once you have some reasonable grasp on what I shall now discuss.

The Concept of Anxiety

The concept of anxiety is central to this whole system of approach. In other words, one might say that anxiety is the general explanatory concept for the interviewee's trying to create a favorable impression. More important, it is this concept which gives the psychiatrist the most general grasp possible on those movements of the patient which mislead him, whether those movements are found in the statements of the informant or in the psychiatrist's interpretation of what he hears. The use of abrupt and accented transitions in the interview becomes understandable in terms of this same concept, for the transitions make it possible for the psychiatrist to alter communicative sets, or to restrain or increase the development of anxiety in the interviewee. And this concept of anxiety can be understood in terms of what everyone of us has known most intimately and continuously from the beginning of our available memory.

An important part of a reasonable grasp on the concept of anxiety might be stated quite simply as: *The presence of anxiety is much worse than its absence*—which is in essence what I have said previously at great length. Under no conceivable circumstance that has ever occurred to me has anyone sought and valued as desirable the experience of anxiety. No series of "useful" attacks of anxiety in therapy will make it something to be sought after. This is, in a good many ways, rather startling, particularly when one compares anxiety with fear. While fear has many of the same characteristics, it may actually be sought out as an experience occasionally, particularly if the fear is expected or anticipated. For instance, people who ride on roller coasters pay money for being afraid. But no one will ever pay money for anxiety in its own right. No one wants to experience it. Only one other experience—that of loneliness—is in this special class of being totally unwanted.

Not only does no one want anxiety, but if it is present, the lessening of it is always desirable, except under the most extraordinary circumstances. Anxiety is to an incredible degree a sign that something ought to be different at once. As the interviewer studies the circumstances of his contact in the interview situation with any stranger, he will observe that those times when the stranger is clearly at a loss to know what the interviewer thinks of him are occasions on which the stranger is suffering considerable anxiety. And anxiety is such a distressing condition to be in that it is often easier for the interviewee to think privately that he is reading the interviewer's mind than to evaluate a situation more realistically. If the interviewer is to have any skill at the work of interrogating, he must realize that he doesn't know what the other fellow is thinking. Yet it is so much more comfortable, even for a psychiatrist, to be carried away by the hope that one does know, that sometimes one acts just as if he did. The only conceivable explanation of this singular travesty of human ability is that it is better than feeling more anxious.

How in the world does it come to be that anxiety exerts such a powerful influence in interpersonal relations? Why does it have this ubiquitous effect of making people act, you might say, like asses? People act so in the exceedingly dubious hope of not being uncomfortable. They may still be terribly uncomfortable when the events are finished, but they haven't suffered as much anxiety as they might have without the use of the defensive behavior. Quite often in the therapy situation, if the patient suffered more anxiety, the returns might be highly desirable. He might not need to experience further anxiety about that particular problem. But that fact makes little difference to the patient. Anxiety rules.

The Development of the Self-System in Personality

It is so extremely important for all of us to maintain any level of euphoria that we are experiencing that we develop a vast system of processes, states of alertness, symbols, and signs of warning, in order to protect what sense of well-being we do have. Although this has its beginning in the relation of the infant and the mothering one, it is first clearly evident in the child as he develops general skills to avoid forbidding gestures; and in the last half of childhood, these skills become elaborated into a great many verbal techniques for putting a somewhat better face on difficult situations. This vast system of operations, precautions, alertnesses, and so on could perfectly properly be called the *self-system*—that part of personality which is born entirely out of the influences of significant others upon one's feeling of well-being. This organization of an enormous number of complex operations comes into existence solely for the purpose of avoiding drops in euphoria which are related to the significant other person with whom the child is integrated. Since these drops in euphoria are, in fact, the same thing as the experience of anxiety, the psychiatrist must realize that every patient carries with him experiences from extraordinarily early in life which make him somewhat cautious about too ready an expression of himself to another by word or gesture. In infancy, we would say that the self-system seeks to protect one's feeling of well-being, of relative euphoria, from a drop in level; and any drop in the sense of well-being is experienced by the infant as anxiety. When we think of the more adult years of existence, it is more informative, more illuminating, to consider the operation of the self-system in terms of operations calculated to protect one's self-esteem; and any lowering of self-esteem is experienced as anxiety. While the formulation is different, we are, in fact, talking about the same thing.

Whether we are talking about infancy or the more adult years of existence, we will speak of these operations for the protection of the self-system as *security operations*. In other words, all anti-anxiety operations are security operations; all efforts to protect one's self-esteem are security operations. It is somewhat easier to see the security element in the processes by which all of us in an adult world practically read into the people around us the movements of our own self-esteem. But I also use the term security operations to refer to the operations of the self-system in the infant, for the adult security operations have their beginnings in the infant's protection of his relative state of euphoria or well-being. One of the great profits that we derive from experience that is well assimilated is better foresight in avoiding unpleasant experience and in gaining good experience. This rather obvious notion about human living can be applied generally to the avoiding of anxiety. Since the other fellow from the beginning to the end has been capable of injuring one's self-esteem, of lowering one's euphoria, it is logical that the self-system should develop into a singularly subtle apparatus for watching for signs of approval and disapproval in the other fellow. But one must remember that the signs that one sees in the other fellow don't necessarily mean too much about him. There is no such thing as "objective" observation; it is participant observation in which you may be the significant factor in the participation.

Thus everybody who comes to the interviewer is very busy interpreting the interviewer while the interviewer is interpreting him. There is some small chance that the interviewer will interpret correctly, but there is little chance that the interviewee will interpret correctly, for the interviewer is not engaged in being anything like a well-rounded person whose durable characteristics would be pertinent to the interview. He is engaged in being an expert at determining what the durable characteristics of the interviewee are. The interviewer's durable characteristics may interfere to some extent with the manifestations of his expert skill in getting a fairly dependable idea of the interviewee. To that extent the interviewer is getting in his own way.

I do not mean to suggest that the perfect interviewer is

opaque and free from meaningful gestures and so on. Were
any one of us to be interviewed about a significant aspect of our
living by a person who gave us no clues as to what he thought
and how we were doing, I think we would be reduced to mut-
ism within a matter of minutes. Our uncertainty would be
frightful, and we would simply be too acutely anxious to go on.
In short, none of us feel that safe, and we won't feel that safe
until the social order has greatly improved in its utility for living. The interviewer actually gives signs by tonal gestures, by
physical gestures, and by verbal statements, which can be, and
are, interpreted and misinterpreted by the interviewee. The
skill in interviewing lies in not doing this in the wrong way.
These gestures and signs of the interviewer may not be greatly
revealing of his ideas regarding the discussion currently in
progress, but they do serve to indicate to the interviewee that
the interviewer is a human being, and that is sufficiently reassuring, makes the interviewee sufficiently comfortable, so that
he is able to go on without getting completely tied up in his uncertainty and anxiety.

Frequently the patient thinks that he has learned just what
impression he is making on the therapist, and gets quite enthusiastic about what he thinks he is conveying to the therapist. The
patient will probably continue to be enthusiastic until a simple
and commonplace question by the therapist shows him that his
concept of the impression he was making was all a mistake. At
this point the patient will experience considerable anxiety. No
matter how painful the experience, the patient often does not
seem to learn anything from it. Having recovered, he may immediately start the cycle over again, building up in his mind
another version of the therapist's impression of him, until it is
interrupted by the therapist and the patient again experiences
anxiety.

In other words, the one thing the therapist can always depend on in psychiatric interviews is that the patient's self-
system will be very active indeed. Unless the interviewee is revealing data bearing on his aptitudes for living, on his successes,
or on his unusual abilities as a human being, the operations of

the self-system are always in opposition to achieving the purpose of the interview. That is, it always opposes the clear revelation of what the interviewee regards as handicaps, deficiencies, defects, and what not, and it does not facilitate communication except in the realms where that which is communicated clearly enhances his sense of well-being, his feeling of making a favorable impression. It is well for the interviewer to calmly assume that this is the way the world is. This is a perduring aspect of reality; it is no cause for lamentation, for contempt of the other fellow, or for irritation at how hard the interviewer has to work for a living. He will then understand that, in his role of participant observer, a very great part of the work of the detailed inquiry is his use of skill to avoid arousing unnecessary anxiety, and at the same time to obtain dependable indices of what the interviewee considers to be significant misfortunes about him, unfortunate incidents in his past, handicaps that he has in dealing with people, and so on. But I trust that I am making it amply clear that the successful psychiatric interview is *not* largely a matter of "showing up" the interviewee.

As I have said, one of the remarkable aspects of the self-system is that after suffering defeat it immediately pulls itself together and goes to work again. This fact has some practical implications for the interviewer's handling of those actions, remarks, processes, and events which are chiefly purposed to protect the self-system of the interviewee. Thus if the interviewer is unduly impressed by the fact that anxiety can be an absolute barrier to interpersonal processes, he may become too "considerate" of the feelings of the interviewee. In that case he will obtain a great deal of data on the manifestations of the interviewee's self-system, but the data won't be of any particular use, for it will do no more than clearly demonstrate that, like all other human beings, the interviewee tries to make a good impression. That discovery will not be enough to solve any problems.

On the other hand, the interviewer may have nothing to do with the interviewee's movements toward reassuring himself, toward putting his best foot forward, but may immediately consign them to oblivion; thus the interviewer precipitates anxiety every time the interviewee tries to avoid it, and the interview becomes unproductive. If the interviewee is a patient, it is perfectly certain he won't return. If he is a candidate for a job, or something of the sort, it is perfectly certain that he will not give the interviewer any adequate basis for forming an opinion.

Now how does one get the data one needs despite the interviewee's anxiety? In the early part of this discourse I laid great stress on the orientation of every interview situation to the achievement of some useful, beneficial effect for the interviewee. I did this with the following in mind: There is a great deal of fairly subtle data to support the notion that every human being, if he has not been tediously demoralized by a long series of disasters, comes fairly readily to manifest processes which tend to improve his efficiency as a human being, his satisfactions, and his success in living—a tendency which I somewhat loosely call *the drive toward mental health*. If one's operations with another person begin to connect with an anticipation on his part of favorable outcome of the experience, then, however unpleasant the details may be, he will begin to be not so immediately deflected by anxiety. If, for example, as a result of very sustained and well-directed efforts on the part of the psychiatrist during three months of intensive therapy, the patient finally sees that the procedure might work, then he will be able to go on despite some increasing anxiety. In fact, if this conviction of favorable change becomes quite strong, the patient will at opportune moments be able to undergo rather rapidly increasing anxiety, even though it may reach a point where his conventional skills are seriously impaired—for example, his speech may be disturbed.

Thus the interviewer, whether he is a psychiatrist or a personnel manager, must learn to facilitate this movement in the interview situation which renders the interviewee's anxiety less immediately deflective—remembering that no intervention, no matter how skillful, can ever render anxiety desirable. When the interviewee's 'tolerance' for anxiety has increased, he can even discuss things that he is quite sure will harm the interviewer's esteem of him.

Remember this, however: The psychiatrist can—if he is both skillful and stupid enough—precipitate intense anxiety and "smash," as some people put it, the patient's defenses; he can "pin him down to the facts," as some have a damnable habit of saying; but he will not get useful information in this way. He will be presented with a great many "phenomena," but there will be no way that he can guess what they are all about. For example, the doctor may feel quite conceited at having brought a patient to the state of practically generalized bodily tremor, whereupon the patient says something like, "Well, Doctor, it really wasn't so. What I actually did was to hit him with an ax." He may have hit somebody with an ax, but when the patient is at that level of anxiety the psychiatrist cannot be sure of anything that he hears. Once in while the beautiful account of the blow with the ax is only a wild guess by the patient as to what the therapist is insisting he must say, and has no particular reference to any other aspects of the patient's past. Anxiety of that intensity puts a terrible strain on the prospects of further results, and gives the psychiatrist data which are useless to him.

But the interviewer does have to deal with anxiety almost eternally. This dealing with anxiety in relations with others is a work of exquisite refinement and crucial importance, at least until the other person sees a high probability that something useful is going to come of it. After that has happened—and the interviewer must be judicious in judging *when* it happens—he may not have to worry quite so much about doing the wrong thing. If he provokes a little anxiety when he doesn't need to, it can usually be assuaged by some sort of mildly reassuring gesture. But until the interviewee becomes convinced that some good will come out of the interview or series of interviews, the psychiatrist must avoid any carelessness about provoking anxiety, or any insensitivity to its manifestations. And he cannot afford to object to the existence of anxiety and its manifestations. To fail in any of these respects is to promote disaster.

Anyone who proceeds without consideration for the disjunctive power of anxiety in human relationships will never learn interviewing. When there is no regard for anxiety, a true interview situation does not exist; instead, there may be just a person (the patient) trying to defend himself frantically from some kind of a devil (the therapist) who seems determined (as the patient experiences it) to prove that the person (the patient) is a double-dyed blankety-blank. This can be a spectacular human performance, but it does not yield psychiatric data relevant to therapeutic progress.

What I have been saying about anxiety and security operations will become more meaningful if you will make a careful study of the next awkward situation that you get into with your boss, your husband or wife, or what not. Needless to say you will only be able to study this awkward situation retrospectively. Although these situations often include various complexities, they are always characterized by anxiety and they always manifest almost simon-pure security operations. That means, of course, that you won't just think about what bright answer you could have made, or something of that kind, but you will actually study all that you can recall of how the situation grew, how you felt, what you did, and so on. Any one of these awkward situations—which, unhappily, most of us have at least one time a day—shows, in microcosm, practically all that anyone needs to really understand about security operations in order to become fairly skillful at provoking them or by-passing them in dealing with other people. When you study particular awkward situations, you may eventually be able to discover that, for instance, a particular remark in a particular tone was what made you feel uncomfortable. This feeling of acute, sort of diffused discomfort is anxiety—however it is experienced, whatever guises and whatever language you attach to it in order to make it feel less unpleasant. The first few times you attempt it—even though you try hard to analyze clearly in your recollection just what went on, one event after another, dealings, thoughts, this and that—you are apt to find that you didn't have any particular discomfort. The other person made you angry, he humiliated you and you were annoyed, you humiliated him—all that sort of thing. But you are then missing completely the thing I am striving to describe—namely, the anxieties that started the fireworks. Until you are able to discover that the first experience in this sequence of events is acute discomfort, you won't make much sense of what I am talking about.

This comes about because anger is much more pleasant to experience than anxiety. The brute facts are that it is much more comfortable to feel angry than anxious. Admitting that neither is too delightful, there is everything in favor of anger. Anger often leaves one sort of worn out, and one thing and another, very often makes things worse in the long run, but there is a curious feeling of power when one is angry. In other words, the expressive pattern of anger tends to drive things away. Not only is anxiety thus avoided, but the initial index of its presence fades from observation, and you are left with no clear idea of how this all came about. In somewhere around 94 per cent of all occasions on which you are anxious, the security operations called out by that anxiety are the things you are perfectly clear on, whereas the precipitating anxiety is obscured.

Discomfort, tense discomfort, a definite sudden transition from fair to worse, a feeling of general ill-being, all of these are of a single genus—they indicate anxiety. It is anxiety which starts you off on the manifestation of these security operations, shown by protesting your rightness, and so on. There are an infinity of ways in which these protective devices, security operations, are displayed. In suggesting that you attempt to notice the movements of premonitory anxiety in yourselves, I am well aware that it will be difficult, if not impossible, to capture the experience of anxiety, since it moves so swiftly into these security operations. But you may be able to discover that in addition to the immediate activation of the security operation, there has been a covert operation which gives you some notion of what in the other person angered you, and so on. You will find that immediately after whatever causes you anxiety you develop an unfavorable estimation of the other person and that you react in response to this. In addition you may discover that the character of your action gives a clear index to the character of your unfavorable appraisal of the person who injured you.

So it is that in interviewing, the interviewer must learn to recognize the anxiety that underlies the security operations in the interviewee. Otherwise he doesn't make very much sense in trying to develop the fairly subtle sensitivity which makes it possible to operate in the field of recurring anxiety with steadily increasing useful results in communication. He studies, by such skills as he can acquire, the indices by which the interviewee indicates his supposition about what the interviewer is thinking. This supposition is the formulated part of what the interviewee thinks he is doing with the interviewer. The interviewer, as he studies these indices, permits the security operations to go on long enough so that he can develop reasonable certainty regarding the sensitivities that called out these security operations—that is, by observing the security operations, he seeks for clues to the location of the underlying anxiety. And when the interviewer has developed a good hunch as to what the insecurity is about, he then tests that hunch by the use of some question designed to suddenly destroy the patient's illusion that he is doing fine in making a good impression. The successive movements in the situation may indicate whether or not the patient is experiencing anxiety, and thus whether the interviewer's hunch was reasonably probable or quite beside the point.

To refer again to your study of your own experience of an awkward situation, you may be able to discover that an acute feeling of ill-being is followed by what looks like two streams of processes. One of these is that you are engaged in some sort of action, often angry action, toward the other person with whom you are involved. The other process, which goes along with the first, is that you are analyzing the situation as one in which this other person has injured you, belittled you, or done something to you which is decidedly unpleasant. If the psychiatrist keeps these processes in mind as he observes his patient, he may notice that the ways in which the patient responds, his angry remarks, and so on, are rather strikingly a revelation of, a communication about, the interpretation that he has made of a particular situation. In other words, if the patient defines a situation as being injurious or anxiety-provoking, what he does shows it. But if the psychiatrist does not recognize that anxiety lies behind the whole performance, he will look in the wrong place for an explanation of the behavior.

Thus the interviewer sees both attempts to make good impressions and angry behavior as security operations which occur under somewhat different circumstances. He observes the pattern of these security operations; he gets some idea about what sort of theory about him, and about the situation, is behind this pattern of activity. He formulates this idea as a hypothesis which must be tested in order to become useful. If he has two hypotheses, all the better, as I have said earlier. In order to test his hypothesis, the interviewer does something designed to disturb the field of operation, and what follows may confirm his hypothesis about where the patient's sensitivity lies. Now, if the hypothesis is correct, none of this is pleasant for the patient, for he ends up with some felt anxiety, unprotected for the moment by his security operation. It is quite important that this should not happen exterior to the interviewer's clear awareness and thus to no useful end. The interviewer must not go through this performance of listening to the interviewee's somewhat rosy account of something, for instance, and then perforate it without trying to learn something from what he is doing. Otherwise the interviewer is manifesting utter disregard and disrespect for the other person concerned, or he is showing an obtuseness, or a deep preoccupation with something else—all of which violates the whole basic notion of the essentially therapeutic or helpful relationship.

It is inevitable that from time to time the interviewer punctures—often very clumsily—the self-esteem of the interviewee. That is all right if the interviewer knows what he is doing, and learns something from it. But if he does it because he is insecure or absent-minded, the detailed inquiry will not develop very satisfactorily. Instead, the interviewer will gather a quite fictitious collection of data about some quite fictitious creature, innocently believed by the interviewer to be the person he is interviewing.

CHAPTER
VI

The Interview as a Process

A GREAT DEAL of our discussion of the interview has suggested that it is a process, or a system of processes—and the word *process* of course implies change. I wish now to present a generalization of this change—that is, a way of looking at it—which will help the interviewer to keep track of what is going on. One kind of change which may go on in the interview situation is *a change in the interviewee's attitude*. A change in the attitude of the other person is fairly easy for anyone to notice in any conversational dealing. But noticing another, equally important group of changes which may occur in an interpersonal situation requires more training, more centered interest. In the interview situation, these somewhat more recondite changes are *changes in the interviewer's attitude, as reflected by the interviewee*. In other words, the interviewer must ask himself: What attitude of mine is being reflected by the interviewee? What does he seem to be experiencing about my attitude? What does he think I am doing? How does he think I feel toward him? A great many useful clues to the complex processes making up the interview first appear when the interviewer begins to think in such terms. Part of his development of skill comes from observing, more or less automatically, what is *probably* the case with respect to the interviewee's feelings about the interviewer's attitude. The interviewee's impression may, of course, be very far from what the interviewer would call "accurate." In other words, even though the interviewer is being highly objective and entirely, respectfully impersonal, it may seem to the interviewee that the interviewer is engaged in showing him up to be no good. The interviewee's operations give clues to what he is experiencing, and in many cases these point toward the type of difficulty that he will have with anyone who impresses him as superior in capability or in position.

Thus it is is quite important to realize that there are two groups of processes directed to the interviewer: one is the *direct attitude* of the interviewee toward him; and the other is that part of the interviewee's performances which are faithfully related to the *supposed attitude* of the interviewer.

Gross Impressions of the Interview Situation

In order to observe change, it is necessary to have some point of departure; and for the detailed inquiry, that point of departure is those gross impressions obtained in the stages of the formal inception and the reconnaissance. The changes from these initial gross impressions which are observed during the later course of the interview are useful as data.

The first rudimentary, gross impression that any interviewer has of a particular interview is in terms of its efficiency: perhaps the interview is "hard going"—that is, the interviewer feels that he really earns his money to get any information at all out of his client; or perhaps the interview is rather "run-of-the-mill," and not in any way unusual; or it may be remarkably productive. It is not difficult to obtain such gross impressions; the interviewer can scarcely avoid noticing it if he must make unusual effort to obtain results, or if, on the other hand, he is required to do very little to gather relevant information. Having obtained this grossest of impressions, he begins to analyze it from several different points of view—and here I will use some popular expressions that point in the direction of what I mean. First he considers the interviewee in terms of his *general alertness*—that is, how keen he is, and in how many areas, and how clearly the implications evoked in his mind of the other person's remarks and questions are related to what might reasonably be expected. In other words, the interviewee's *attention* to what is going on may vary greatly. Some people are *intent* on everything the interviewer says, and are very careful about everything they produce, but at the same time are not guarded; they are simply determined to get something out of the interview. There are others who are *distracted;* noises outside, or things that are going on in their own minds, get in the way of their following closely the questions, comments, and suggestions of the interviewer. Occasionally a person's attention in the interview situation may be appropriately called *vague.* Such people seem to have only the most casual and foggy contact with what the interviewer is trying to get at, and the responses that they produce seem to have at best a tenuous or nebulous relationship to what the other person has said.

Along with all this, the interviewer develops an impression of the *"intelligence"* of the interviewee. First impressions of the intelligence of another person can be quite misleading. For example, every now and then in employment interviewing one encounters a person who literally doesn't seem to know the language. Inquiry into his employment history, however, may show that he has made extremely rapid progress in handling complex machinery in an industrial job, and the interviewer realizes that to have done this he must have very high general intelligence. Thus one must always realize that intelligence, in the sense of something which is useful as an aid in living, is by no means necessarily measurable by verbal dexterity. Verbal dexterity is closely related to intelligence only if there has been opportunity for the development of verbal skills.

Finally, in this group of very general characteristics, the interviewer may notice the *responsiveness* of the interviewee. People who are quite responsive—a very broad term in the sense that I use it here—are apt to be commended by their friends as having a peculiarly "sensitive understanding"; that is, they are likely to be sufficiently sensitive to such things as minor tonal indices so that they are able with a minimum of awkward questions to catch on to those things which are embarrassing for other people to communicate. Responsiveness includes a group of complex elements in the personality which, other things being equal, make for ease in living, and which in their very highest manifestation, perhaps, add up to what is ordinarily called "tact." In the interview situation, the responsiveness of the interviewee can vary from *understanding cooperation*, in which he almost knows what the next question will be, and provides a succinct and illuminating answer as soon as it is asked, to an *obtuseness* such that he gets completely lost trying to guess what the interviewer is driving at, apparently deriving very little from those indications that would suffice for an "understanding" person. Sometimes obtuseness seems to border on something that is probably hostile; in other words, there are people whose dumbness is all but deliberate. Sometimes there is a certain *unwillingness to be led*, so that it is singularly difficult to get the interviewee to deal with the topics that one presents, although he may be very productive about something quite irrelevant, or about something that is important but tangential at the moment. Occasionally there are interviewees—sometimes court cases, sometimes difficult children—who are, the interviewer is apt to think, *deliberately obstructive*. It clearly seems that such an interviewee is engaged in trying to prevent the interviewer's getting his points across, and is attempting to keep anything of interest from the interviewer.

These are only hints of the kinds of gross impressions that the interviewer has gathered by the time he begins the detailed inquiry; such gross impressions, which may, of course, be wrong, form the point of departure from which he observes change.[1]

---

[1] [*Editors' note:* This chapter is taken from the 1945 series of lectures. In his 1944 lecture on the same topic, Sullivan mentioned two other gross impressions which the interviewer may obtain, which he described as "related to the elaboration of observation rather than to observation itself":

"It is useful to note the patient's *habitual attitude toward his recall or memory*. Recall is a function of motivation, and the person's attitude toward his own recall—be it assurance, vague uncertainty, or emphatic pessimism— may be quite revealing. By an attitude of assurance, I do not mean that anyone knows that his memory will always work, for nobody's memory always works. I, for example, find it extremely difficult to recall ordinal data—names of telephone exchanges, names of people, and so on and so forth—but I usually recall anything which I need badly, and so my attitude toward my recall function is rather trusting. I expect it to work if there is a reasonable cause for it to do so; however, I don't expect to be able to remember poetry, for instance, since, so far as I know, it will never be useful to me. In contrast, there are people who almost always wonder if what they recall from the

He realizes, of course, that at the same time that he is picking up these gross impressions of the interviewee, the interviewee is picking up gross impressions of him. Thus it is quite rewarding for the interviewer to be curious about those signs in the remarks and performances of the interviewee which reflect to the interviewer the sort of person that the interviewee surmises him to be.

I would now like to mention some of the more specific terms which are used quite frequently by the interviewer to describe

year before last is right or wrong. They don't seem to have any particular optimism as to their success at recalling anything; they simply don't trust their recollection. I think that most of these people don't mention this distrust; it is something they don't brag about. On the other hand, when you encounter someone who talks about how rotten his memory is, the chances are that he *does* trust it—and that you can't trust his statements. Thus the interviewer can make some estimate of the patient's recall. Is what he has lived through handy to him, available to him when he needs it? Or are many matters of the past to be looked upon as lost, strayed, or stolen? It is not that recall is important in itself, but that the person's *attitude* toward recall gives a valuable clue to the simplicity of his motivation. If his recall is relatively useful to him, he has probably been proceeding toward more or less clearly foreseen goals for a long time, and having some success at getting nearer them; and his motivational system is relatively simple. In trying to trace some unhappy people's motivational history, one may get into quagmires which take hours to wallow through, whereas one could have found a useful and immediate clue to much the same thing by noticing to what extent they could depend on their memories.

"An inference can also be made in regard to the patient's *habitual feeling about answering questions.* Some people are at an atrocious disadvantage with almost anybody if they are put in the position of answering questions; and no matter how suavely one handles the interview, such people will soon discover that they are being required to answer a lot of questions, and will feel this very keenly. This attitude reflects certain things about the interviewee's past, but it also gives the interviewer a fairly important hunch as to how much faster things will proceed if he can only get this person to talking about things, so that the interviewer can be quiet and listen, only coming in now and then with a conversational remark. Of course, if time is very limited and the problem is very complex, one can scarcely have recourse to this. Under such circumstances, when somebody goes into a mild upset because a question is flung at him, one can sometimes, believe it or not, diminish the evil effects by saying, 'Do you feel I'm questioning you?' At that, any completely sane person would say quite angrily, 'I *know* you are questioning me!' But people who are upset are so glad to have anything that looks like a straw thrown to them that they don't notice the preposterous character of such an inquiry, and actually feel better about what the interviewer is doing, having somehow slipped away from the anxiety connected with being questioned."]

the interviewee, and which provide a somewhat more refined impression of the processes that go on to make up the interview. The following sets of attitudes suggest patterns which the interviewer will use as starting points in observing change in his relation with the interviewee. While these are words of common speech, I also hope to have them carry some fairly specific meaning. In the early stages of the interview, the interviewee may seem to be, for example, *reserved, guarded, suspicious, hostile,* or *contemptuous.* A quite different set of five terms may also characterize the same interviewee from a somewhat different standpoint: his manner toward the interviewer may be *supercilious, superior, conciliatory, deferential,* or *apologetically inferior.* There are two situations which may be presented by the interviewee in the early stages of his work which are of peculiar difficulty, and for that reason it is very important for an interviewer to consider carefully how to deal with them. One is presented by the *insolent informant;* in certain types of interview work the informant may be thoroughly insolent— and it is nice indeed when this changes. Something which is much more common in psychiatric work, and also quite common in all other forms of interviewing, is the situation presented by the *evasive informant.*

The Observation of Changes in the Interview Situation

The interviewer's interest is in observing the *changes* that appear in such sets of attitudes—in observing what in the situation is improving or what is deteriorating. Sometimes, of course, it is the impression of the interviewer that there is little or no change. Perhaps during the inception of the interview and the reconnaissance the interviewer has, as nearly as he can judge, developed impressions of the interviewee which are fairly accurate. Perhaps the interviewee began as a somewhat supercilious person. As the interviews progress, he still sounds as if he thought the interviewer were one of the very great headaches that it had been his misfortune to encounter; there isn't a bit of change. These situations in which there seems to be no particular alteration in the attitude of the informant in the course of a well-conducted interview are highly significant, for reasons which I trust I shall be able to make clear a little later. Sometimes, of course, the psychiatrist sees a *mutually respecting* person—one who shows such obvious self-respect, and therefore respect for the other person, that the interviewer has the feeling, "Well, bless us! What on earth does this man need of a psychiatrist?" Sometimes the answer is that these people are not seeking cures, but are seeking jobs or something else, for the interview is used for many purposes besides finding cures. A fairly clearly self-respecting attitude, with respect also shown for the other person—the one does not exist without the other —is not likely to undergo very much change during an interview or series of interviews unless the interviewer very seriously disappoints the person who possesses it.

Besides noting change, and having some idea of what that change is, in terms of what is improved, what is deteriorated, or what has shown no change at all, the interviewer tries to pick up, more or less automatically, impressions of what in his own performance has had some bearing on the change. If the situation is bad—the interview is hard going for some reason or other—it is well for the interviewer to have some idea as to what operations of his are responsible for the failure to produce any change, even though he may have thought they were well adjusted to improving the situation. If he knows what he was trying to do, and if he is able to study—in the interstices of other things, as it were—how well he did it, how flatly it failed, or how dramatically it succeeded, then he will have important data related to the motivational system which characterizes the interviewee.

As I have already suggested, the interviewer will have a gross impression of the informant's changing impression of the interviewer, as shown by the informant's attitude. There are in this field three areas, if you please, of major importance. First, the interviewer may ask himself: Is the patient being impressed with the therapist's *expertness in interpersonal relations?* Second: Is the patient coming more and more to appreciate the therapist as an *understanding person?* That is, whether the therapist is friendly or austere, does he show an interest in sparing the informant's "feelings"—or, more accurately, does he pay as much respect as possible to the informant's need to feel self-esteem? As an indication of what I mean by "understanding," consider a situation in which a therapist, for some reason or other, is interviewing a seventeen-year-old about the details of his sex life. Some interviewers would ask blunt questions, which might serve the purpose of giving the adolescent some new ideas about possible sexual ventures which had not occurred to him before, but would usually have the main result of producing such anxiety that the adolescent would not even be able to stutter, and nothing useful would go on, either visibly or audibly. Other interviewers in such a situation would be so careful that unhappily they would not get any useful information either; even though they thought they did, further inquiry would show that they did not. Thus the really understanding person is not so tender to the interviewee that he prevents his doing what he is there for, but he does not make it any more distressing than he can help, even though he may seem very cold and remote. The third major question about the patient's impression of the interviewer is this: Does he seem to feel a *simplicity of motivation* in the therapist—that the therapist is solely interested in doing a competent job? In other words, to what extent does the patient seem to consider that the therapist is concerned primarily with getting valid data from which to reach valid conclusions about him and his troubles; and to what extent does he seem to think that the therapist is activated by ulterior motives?

Assessing changes in these areas is important. Insofar as the patient seems to be more and more impressed by the doctor's expert skill, and more and more relieved by his understanding way of doing things, and perfectly convinced that the doctor has no objective except finding out who the patient is, and what ails him—to that extent the serious work of the interview is being vastly expedited, and the difficulties in the patient's personality will be increasingly presented with a minimum of wear and tear on the doctor. When these impressions are not so favorable, the data are presented in such a way as to make their interpretation more difficult, since there is less freedom of movement in the interpersonal field—that is, the patient's ability to express himself is more restricted.

Impressions as Hypotheses To Be Tested

These gross impressions that I am talking about are, in fact, rough hypotheses, and, like all hypotheses in interpersonal work, they should be subjected to continuous, or recurrent, test and correction. Sometimes the interviewer is able, almost as automatically as a calculating machine, to add up negative and positive evidence of this and that so that he simply knows, without any particularly laborious thinking, that the patient is, let us say, improving. In such a case, the interviewer has so continuously and automatically tested his hypotheses that he knows the answer without bothering to do anything about it very consciously or deliberately.

But more frequently the interviewer obtains impressions which on scrutiny may or may not be justifiable. More or less specific testing operations should be applied to those impressions with the idea of getting them more nearly correct. One way these impressions are tested is by more or less *unnoted inference*. However, the testing of hypotheses cannot safely be left wholly to relatively unformulated referential operations. Instead it is well for the interviewer now and then to think about the impressions that he has obtained. The very act of beginning to formulate them throws them into two rough groups: *those about which one has no reasonable doubt* and *those which, when noted, are open to question.* The latter, of course, need further testing. A so-called "highly intuitive" interviewer who does not formulate his impressions, but relies solely on his unnoted inference, is likely to find that after an interview is over some most pregnant questions arise in his mind —and he has failed to secure any clues whatever to the answers. That is the danger if one depends on the machinery outside of awareness to do all the work, instead of attempting now and then to take stock of one's impressions. The other way of testing hypotheses is by *clearly purposed exploratory activity* of some kind. The interviewer asks critical questions—that is, questions so designed that the response will indicate whether the hypothesis is reasonably correct or quite definitely not adequate.

The Situation of Improving Communication

Let us consider now the general case in which the interview situation shows, more or less continuously, or at least from period to period, definitely improving communication. This is the situation in which everything is going well. For the inexperienced interviewer, that can be a great misfortune, for he may fail to notice carefully and as completely as possible all of the context—the operations, the remarks, and their patterns—which lead to distinct improvements in the situation. If the interviewer knows how the situation came to be going so well, in the sense that he knows at which points of his operations the patient's communicability increased, he has quite valuable indices to the informant's covert security operations—that is, his security operations which are only inferentially evident. In other words, the interviewer can find, in the context that led to distinct improvements in the interviewee's freedom of communication, fairly clear grounds for inferring what sort of thing led him to suffer anxiety; improvement in the patient's communication at a particular time implies that the patient at that time experienced relief from the feeling that he would make a bad impression, give away something disastrous, or something of the sort. Looking back a little further, the interviewer can then begin to see the general pattern of the interviewee's precautions, the security operations by which he was guarding some particular area until the interviewer did something that made it seem safe to go ahead.

Thus, unless the interviewer pays close attention to the more or less episodic improvements in the interview that goes "wonderfully," he may miss a great deal of the data that might show what the interviewee would be like in a more difficult situation that didn't go so smoothly. The same things are to be found out about the interviewee in the interviews that go well as in the interviews that go badly, but in the first instance they are revealed only if the interviewer notices each favorable change, and thinks of it in terms of what the patient was doing earlier, which has now been made unnecessary.

The Situation of Deteriorating Communication

Now let us consider the special case in which deterioration of the communicative attitude is occurring: the patient is getting less communicative and acts as though he thought that the interviewer were anything but an expert. When things seem to be going from bad to worse, I should counsel any therapist to control his anxiety for the moment, if possible, and to try to study the deterioration in the relationship by retrospective survey, for a great deal may be gained in this way. (I trust that it is becoming clear why I emphasize that it is well for the interviewer to have some recall of what has gone on—which is unlikely if he simply shoots out questions as fast as he can, ignoring the answers.) The interviewer may begin this study by trying to sort out the time when deterioration first seemed to characterize the relationship. Sometimes a psychiatric interview goes badly from the inception, from the time the interviewer uttered his first remarks to the stranger. More often, the bad going begins during the reconnaissance. Perhaps the interviewer, by his way of getting the gross social history of the patient, has fallen over some security apparatus of the patient —and if this is so, it is a very good thing to know. Or in retrospect the interviewer may realize that the inception of the interview was characterized by a certain willingness and mutual regard on the part of both, that they got through the reconnaissance or outline of social history quite well, and that actually for some time in the detailed inquiry everything seemed to be quite all right—until at a certain point the interviewer asked something, the patient replied, and events seemed to go sour thereafter. Such a discovery is very useful indeed, both as a basis for rectifying the deteriorating situation and, much more important, as data for achieving the purpose of the interview. Things don't have to be lovely for an interview to succeed; some quite unpleasant interviews may give the interviewer a pretty good impression of what ails the other fellow. I might add that the longer the interviewer has been working with a particular person, the more possible it is to be reasonably certain of what did happen. Early in a relationship, the interviewer may know what *he* said, and he may know what *the patient* said; but nevertheless it was as if two strangers were talking to themselves. Later interviews often progress to what amounts to singularly subtle communications of fact. The longer the relationship has gone on, the greater is the possibility of the interviewer's being reasonably certain of just when things went wrong, and what was probably the situation at the time deterioration appeared.

In considering this question of timing, the interviewer should note whether the situation began going from bad to worse insidiously or relatively abruptly. If its appearance was relatively abrupt, careful review in the interviewer's own mind of the apparent circumstances will give him a hunch as to what was the matter, and this hunch can then be tested in various ways. If in retrospect the interviewer cannot determine any particular time at which things seemed to get worse, but feels that matters have been getting worse insidiously from the beginning, he has something on his hands which may be quite intricate. In this case, *first*, he may well *review the factual basis for his earlier more favorable appraisal of the situation*. Sometimes he may discover in retrospect that his own enthusiasm, rather than that of the patient, was responsible for his feeling that things had been better in the beginning. In other words, in some supposedly insidiously deteriorating situations, matters have been very bad from the beginning, and the patient has been more and more driven to impress upon the interviewer how bad things are, until the interviewer finally catches on. But that is not deterioration. When the interviewer grasps the fact that the situation is bad, that is, if anything, a slightly favorable change, since communication has improved. Thus it is well to look back to see whether there was any valid reason for thinking that things were once going better and now are going worse.

Second, and this is very important in the situation which really is deteriorating, the interviewer should review what has happened as best he can to *learn whether anything discouraging as to the outcome of the interview has occurred.* Has the interviewer said or seemed to imply something, or encouraged the patient to say something (which the interviewer has not neutralized) which discourages the patient's hope of a useful outcome of the interview? When a person loses heart about an interpersonal relation, things begin to be dull, and the person tends to think about how to get out of it politely. Most psychiatrists have had this unpleasant retrospective realization that they have said, or have permitted the patient to say without rejoinder, something which is seriously discouraging. After that things may go much worse. In some instances, the patient is so far ahead of the psychiatrist that he soon realizes that things are not going to work with this particular psychiatrist, and so, practically from the start, he is thinking about how he can escape and try it with someone else.

Third, it is well for the interviewer who is looking for the facts about a deteriorating interview situation to *observe what relation the current situation has to his own attitude toward this interviewee.* He should consider what his attitude has been from the start, or what it has been since some particular event —for example, perhaps the interviewee said something which displeased the interviewer, or which caused a sudden concentration of the interviewer's interest. Sometimes the young doctor finds data about mother, and father, and maiden aunts, and so on, rather boring and uninspiring, but gets greatly interested in some "problem" such as masturbation—and sometimes interview situations deteriorate lamentably after such a sudden evincing of unexpected interest on the part of the doctor. Thus when things are deteriorating rather insidiously, it is well for the interviewer to check up on whether he took a dislike to this patient when he came in; whether the patient offended the interviewer in some way; or whether, unfortunately, the interviewer showed undue interest in some aspects of the data in such a way that the intelligent patient could interpret it as meaning that the interviewer was very little interested in him, but was interested in some aspect of life of which he happened to be the present entertaining example.

I now want to mention several further attitudes which may appear as changes in the interview, either on the part of the interviewer or the interviewee. Let us consider particularly the situations in which the informant becomes *bored*, is definitely *amused* at an inquiry by the interviewer, is clearly *irritated*, or is frankly *angry*. Changes in the interview situation represented by the appearance of any of these attitudes on the part of the patient are none too cheering. These same attitudes may, of course, appear in the interviewer; on occasion some of them may be deliberately assumed by the interviewer. There are times when it is well for the interviewer to express boredom, mild amusement, or even irritation; however, if the interviewer is genuinely angry, I would say that this is probably tantamount to a serious defect in his equipment for interviewing. Then there are patients who are from the beginning, or become at some later stage in the work, *frivolous*, *flippant*, *arrogant*, *insolent*, *sarcastic*, or *ironic*. On the part of the interviewer, there are occasionally circumstances, if the interviewer is sufficiently expert, in which it may be useful for him to express any except the first two and the last of these attitudes. So far as I know, a frivolous attitude is never under any circumstances useful on the part of an interviewer. I also very firmly disadvise the least flippancy under any circumstances—and that applies with all the greater force to dealings with the patient who begins interview situations flippantly. Patterning one's activities after the informant in that case leads to distinctly less than nothing. And an ironic attitude by the interviewer is often wasted and may cause a lot of trouble; for irony, if at all subtle, may easily be misleading and may get one into rather inextricable situations. Thus I warn the interviewer against being ironic.

Informants at times show rather abrupt changes by becoming decidedly more evasive than they have been up to that time.

Occasionally they become quite *actively obstructive;* they insist emphatically on talking beside the point, so that the interviewer can scarcely overlook the definite unwillingness to follow him and to deal with what he considers to be urgent. Especially in the psychiatric field, the interviewer encounters every now and then a patient who grows, the interviewer feels quite sure, *obscurely suspicious.*

These attitudes which I have now named are all rather important indices to change in the interview situation. I shall try to be a little more informative later on, but at present I am trying to build a sort of very rough fence on which we may or may not be able to grow a few vines later. Let me now present a rule which the interviewer might well engrave somewhere on his interior: *All through the interview process, even in the terminating phases, it is important for the interviewer to covertly verify his observations; he must not merely automatically, perhaps unwittingly, "react" to the patient's expressed attitudes, whether by tone, by gesture, or by words.* All of us are very prone to the automatic response—in fact, life is so exceedingly complex that we need a great many ways of handling things on the spur of the moment—but this has very little place in the intensely complex and therefore rather extraordinarily uncertain work of the psychiatric interview. While the appearance of spontaneity is desirable in the interviewer's responses to affective movements and changes in the patient, these responses should never be automatic in the way they might be with his wife, or his child, or the bus driver, for in the very act of the automatic response, selective inattention probably eliminates about half of the useful data. No interviewer can afford this.

The Theorem of Reciprocal Emotion

Now let me shift to a somewhat more theoretical consideration of the matters which I have been discussing. As I have already indicated, the interview is a system, or a series of systems, of *interpersonal processes,* arising from participant observation in which the interviewer derives certain conclusions about the interviewee. Under these circumstances, interview situations fall under a general principle which I have organized as the *theorem of reciprocal emotion*. That theorem is as follows: Integration in an interpersonal situation is a process in which (1) complementary needs are resolved (or aggravated); (2) reciprocal patterns of activity are developed (or disintegrated); and (3) foresight of satisfaction (or rebuff) of similar needs is facilitated.

This theorem is an extremely general statement which, thus far in my explorations, has seemed to have no serious defects. I believe that if one studies its full implications, a great many things pertaining to the study of interpersonal relations, and pertaining to the participant observation by which the interviewer gets his data, will be clarified. In this general statement, I use the word "needs" in the broadest sense, in the generic sense. Thus, in discussing the development of personality, we speak of all the important motives, or "motors," of human behavior as *needs for satisfaction*. There is a *need* for satisfaction of various forces such as lust and hunger; and *need* in this particular sense also includes the need for a feeling of personal security in interpersonal relations, which in turn can be called a need to avoid, alleviate, or escape from anxiety, or, again, a need for self-esteem.

Now, I have stated, in the first part of the theorem, that complementary needs may be resolved, and reciprocal patterns of activity developed. For example, in the realm of security operations, the urge to reassure is complementary to the need for reassurance. Reassuring by implication, instead of by direct praise or direct reassurance, is the pattern of activity which is reciprocal to the pattern, in the other person, of discounting or inverting direct praise or appreciation. In other words, if a person must discount, disbelieve, or convert into its opposite, all direct praise, then the reciprocal pattern of activity which would appear in a simple interpersonal situation would be reassurance by implication—by saying something which would have very little to do directly with the other person's self-esteem, but would, on further elaboration, be seen to imply a favorable view or hopeful outlook. The experience of an interpersonal situation thus characterized—that is, characterized by such complementary needs and reciprocal patterns of action—tends toward its future reintegration (that is, its recurrence), on the basis of either witting or unnoted anticipation of improvement of one's self-esteem in or by the relationship.

This is a very general pattern of thinking about all interpersonal relations. Now I wish to show how this general pattern may bear on interview situations. Let us consider an interview situation in which the *interviewer* communicates—by tonal gestures, or by the pattern of his remarks, or both, which is usually the case—*his own* need for reassurance. The most common way in which interviewers show their need for reassurance is not by asking for it, but by some form of activity which is calculated to "score off," disparage, belittle, or humiliate the patient in the course of the interview. In fact, such activities, almost without exception, really express a need of the interviewer for some reassurance as to his importance, however dimly the patient may realize this. In this case, the need in the patient which would be complementary, and therefore lead to resolution, would be a somewhat curious thing: a need to be despised. As a matter of fact, there actually are situations in which it is perfectly reasonable to say that a person needs to be despised. However, this is quite a novelty in security needs, and is not likely to occur in the psychiatric interview. In fact, it could really occur in the psychiatric interview only as a complex motive addressed to a goal quite exterior to that of the ordinary interview situation. I can suggest an example of it in another situation, however: A number of our OSS agents accomplished very good work toward winning the war by supplying in their behavior a clear expression of a "need to be despised," as a result of which people in need of this type of reassurance became quite free with them, and gave away things that the agents needed to find out. But these were not interview situations, in the sense that I am discussing them. The OSS men were really the interviewers and not the interviewees, but their informants, in making them the victims of their contempt, fortunately mistook their roles. One does not expect this to happen in successful psychiatric interviews.

Now what does happen in the psychiatric interview if the

interviewer expresses a need to be reassured by lording it over his victim? I have said that, by cultural definition, the patient is the client of an expert, and therefore is inferior in significant respects. Because in this situation he feels himself less capable, he must need reassurance by the performance of the interviewer. Consequently (and this follows the first part of my theorem), the need of the interviewer himself to be reassured is not met by a complementary need on the part of the interviewee, and thus the interviewee's need for security, instead of being resolved, is *aggravated*. To take up the second part of my theorem: If the interviewee is to develop a pattern of activity which is *reciprocal* to the interviewer's pattern, this must be a pattern of submissive or other interviewer-reassuring activity. Or, if he does not develop such a pattern, the communicative activity is *disintegrated*—the thing breaks up.

The development by the interviewee of this reciprocal pattern of a submissive attitude represents an unfortunate situation. If in the development of the interview relation, the interviewee gets the impression that he must have certain views to please the interviewer, and proceeds to submit to this demand, from then on the data that the interviewer gets will be practically beyond interpretation. Unless the interviewer is extremely clever at interpreting interpersonal data, he will make nothing, except what he reads into it, out of the information which the submissive informant dutifully gives him. The interviewer will get a very poor picture of the informant, in comparison with the picture that, for example, an esteemed neighbor would have of him. This is a very poor result for a psychiatric inquiry to have, and so the interviewer, if he is at all skillful at interpreting very complex situations, will not permit the interviewee to fall into one of these submissive relationships in the first place.

And finally, to apply the last part of my theorem: In this situation, the interviewee will develop an alert foresight of the rebuff of his implied need for reassurance, and this will make it certain that he will protect his self-esteem. That is, the longer such a situation goes on, the more he is governed by the foresight of any indication that there will be an aggravation of his anxiety. Since his anxieties are always detestably unpleasant and a potent driving force to get him away from that which causes them, he becomes more and more careful that none of his insecurities are advertised to the security-needing interviewer.

The Patterns of Outcome of Interpersonal Situations

The interpersonal processes making up the interview follow the general pattern of all interpersonal processes, which can be illustrated by a diagram:

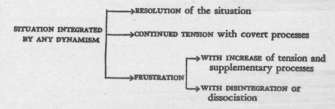

A situation integrated by any dynamism—for example, lust or the pursuit of security—manifests processes which result in one of three subsequent situations: First, there may be a resolution of the situation. For example, the waitress may say, "Do you want cherry or banana pie?" When the customer says, "Banana," that resolves the situation. And in all other situations, the simple, delightful, and final outcome of an interpersonal configuration is that it is resolved: all tension connected with it is washed up, and the thing is finished until something provokes a similar situation.

The second possibility is that a situation may be continued with tension and with covert processes. In this case the person goes on doing the same thing, more or less covertly, but he also begins *to think*, whether noted or unnoted. In other words, he begins to look around for what is wrong, to discover what can be done to effect a satisfactory resolution.

The third possibility is that the processes in the situation may lead to what we call *frustration*. There are two possible states subsequent to frustration. One is marked by an *increase of tension*, reflecting the need which was concerned, and by *supplementary processes*, which may range all the way from circus movements to exceedingly skillful ways of circumventing the obstacles, so that there is a belated resolution of the situation. Sometimes the psychiatrist must deal with situations in which he knows that any frontal attack, any direct approach, would lead to complete frustration. Thus he devises supplementary processes that will weave around the blocking anxiety, so that finally the patient, feeling reasonably secure, will arrive at a point which could never be approached frontally. The other outcome of frustration may be *disintegration of the dynamism* itself and the whole motivational system, or *dissociation*—and processes in interviews involving dissociation are very complex.

The Interviewer's Use of the Foregoing Formulations

I have now tried to set up two very general considerations: (1) that all interview situations fall under the theorem of reciprocal emotion, and (2) that the processes in interview situations follow this general pattern of all interpersonal processes. From these two relatively broad considerations, it follows that the interviewer shows his skill in his choice of a passive or active role at particular junctures in the interview. He may work successfully in a deteriorating situation *if it is not permitted to disintegrate*. Sometimes working in a deteriorating situation is unavoidable; sometimes it is desirable. In general, however, other things being equal, he secures best results most economically in a situation that is improving.

At awkward moments, the interviewer's inquiry progresses from expressed puzzlement to direct questions and, if necessary, finally to the use of "as if." For example, the psychiatrist may tell the patient that he gets the impression that the patient is acting "as if" the psychiatrist had done so-and-so; and then he sees what happens. In any case, he attends respectfully to anything that seems to be communicatively "intended" in the way of answers and comments. If he can make nothing of a remark of the patient's, or if it seems irrelevant, he seeks to re-call the earlier context of the interviews, which may be what it relates to. He does not hesitate to take "time out" for this review; he may be silent for a while before pushing further. If he finds nothing from this hurried looking-back which gives what the patient has said any meaning or relevance, he pauses perhaps momentarily to decide whether it is important; there is a good deal that does not actually deserve any particular further inquiry. But if it does seem that the matter might be important, then the interviewer tries to find out about it. He may take a chance by asking some question about it, and as a result the patient may be able to correct him emphatically. As I have said before, often a great deal of real illumination is gained when the interviewer expresses something which is clearly wrong and the informant puts him right. Somehow, there is a curious relaxation when the interviewee has a chance to correct the interviewer, and at such a juncture the interviewee usually tells a good deal more than he had intended. In fact, my own experi-ence in psychotherapy has been that the occasions when pa-tients have been able to correct my errors—for example, about their histories or about what had moved them in some situation —have been fully as valuable as any equal space of time I have ever spent doing anything else. Sometimes, of course, it is useful for the therapist to deal with a remark that he does not under-stand by simply saying, "I am not sure that I follow. Will you say it another way?" In this way he avoids committing any errors in the asking of his question.

When I spoke earlier of anger, I suggested that anger is not one of the attitudes which an interviewer is permitted to expe-rience toward the interviewee. I trust that this is an absolutely, completely, explicit statement: *anger, in either its mild or severe grades, is one of the most common masking operations for anxiety*. The interviewer may "use" signs of mild irritation or even expressions of anger, but if he is actually angry, that usu-ally means that he himself is in need of some psychotherapeutic help, either from himself or from someone else. It is impossible for an interviewer who really loses his temper now and then with his informant to meet the very technical needs of interviewing and to obtain anything like dependable conclusions.

On the other hand, anxiety is scarcely to be avoided by any interviewer, at least in the course of some few of the interviews which make up his work. Even an interviewer with twenty-five or thirty years of experience will certainly, particularly if he interviews incipient psychotics, be very acutely anxious in his work now and then. And when the interviewer is inexperienced, it is often a question as to whether he or the interviewee has the most anxiety.

Skill in interviewing includes, as a very great part of its basis, certain *processes* for so dealing with occasions of anxiety that the work of the interview is not seriously impaired. There are two statements which I can make about these processes which save the interview situation from the anxiety which the interviewer is bound to experience now and then in his work. *First*, the interviewer should *be alert* to the minor movements of anxiety "in himself" so that he can exercise foresight with respect to the processes which follow. In almost everyone, a great deal of anxiety occurs of which the person concerned has no clear awareness. Some supplementary process such as irritation or anger is rushed onto the scene, and only the most careful retrospective search could give a hint that there was anxiety. In the interview situation, instead of getting away from anxiety as quickly as possible, the interviewer must pay great attention to the movement as he experiences it. If he avoids it, somehow "ignores" that anxiety, he will not learn from it. By observation of those events to which the anxiety is related, the interviewer may learn, not only about himself, but also about the relationship with his patient. Anxiety is unpleasant, but since its experience is inevitable, it should not be lightly cast aside as an ally.

Second, the interviewer should attempt to *identify the seeming cause* of the anxiety. By "seeming" I imply that such "cause" may be quite simply an incipient rationalization—and it will do no harm for the interviewer to recognize this possibility. In looking for the cause, the interviewer may first consider the interviewee as a source of reflected esteem. If the therapist feels that his esteem is falling in the eyes of his patient, he then has the task of exploring whether this is so, and if it is, the reasons for this shift in position.

The next step is to consider the possibility that the anxiety arises in reference to the therapist's supposed failure to live up to what he imagines is the patient's ideal, although this ideal might scarcely be within the effective knowledge of the actual patient. Thus the therapist might "observe himself being a therapist" in comparison with what he imagines is the behavior of Dr. A, some more or less distinguished colleague. In such a comparison the therapist may feel "inferior" and suffer anxiety. Here he may ask a simple question: What is there in the relationship between the therapist and the patient that at this juncture leads the therapist to entertain daydreams concerning his supposed comparison with a colleague?

Last, in looking for the seeming cause of the anxiety, the interviewer may ask if it has some reference to a *foreseen* development—something that will or may happen. The possibilities of this suspected future event may usefully be studied, the anxiety having served a somewhat indirect but important purpose in attracting attention to the possible developments.

In any case, anxiety in the interviewer cannot be entirely avoided; it is clear indication, at least, that he is quite human. Since it will be with him at times, he might as well make use of it. That he can only do by observing it as best he can.

CHAPTER
VII

The Developmental History
as a Frame of Reference in the
Detailed Inquiry

I HAVE SUGGESTED that it is very important indeed for the interviewer to pay attention to anxiety, particularly his own anxiety. Anxiety is of such overwhelming and all but ubiquitous significance in the understanding of interpersonal relations that it is helpful to keep in mind during the entire interview a two-part schematization of the hypothetical personality of the interviewee, which the interviewer is trying to formulate. This two-part schematization—which, like every abstract scheme, is misleading if you take it too literally—is a useful way for the interviewer to organize his thinking. According to this, the personality is divided into (1) the *self-system* and (2) *the 'rest'* of the personality.

The interviewer is always in contact with this self-system of the interviewee. If I have made any sense in my comments to you about anxiety, you must realize that whenever you are dealing with a stranger, both you and the stranger are very seriously concerned with matters of appraisal, of esteem, respect, deference, prestige, and so on, and that all of these are manifestations of the self-system. The protection of these matters is the very reason for the existence of the self-system. Therefore the one thing you can always be sure of is that it is a rare moment indeed in an interview situation, however prolonged, in which the self-system of the interviewee is not centrally concerned.

This means that all through the development of the interview situation, however prolonged, the interviewee is showing efforts to avoid, minimize, and conceal signs of his anxiety from the interviewer and from 'himself' [1]—that is, in a certain locution, keeping himself from *knowing* that he is anxious. In other words, the concealment applies both to the interviewer and to the person interviewed. But that is to some extent a figure of speech rather than a precise statement; that is, people conceal their anxiety from themselves and others by the promptness with which they do something about it.

The interviewee's self-system is at all times, but in varying degrees, in opposition to achieving the purpose of the interview. This is an elaborate but fairly correct way of saying what might be said casually as: The self-system of the stranger is always viewing the other person as an enemy and taking due precautions against the other person on that basis. The interviewer's skill, therefore, addresses itself to circumventing the interviewee's security operations without increasing the scope or the subtlety of these operations. The amateur interviewer, in trying to circumvent the anxiety of the interviewee, may make the manifestations of the security operations more subtle so that they won't disturb him. Thus the interviewer must have skill in order to avoid this calling out of more security operations or more obscure and subtle ones. This, in effect, amounts to the interviewer's avoiding unnecessary provocation of anxiety without at the same time missing data which are needed for a reasonably correct assessment of the person with whom he is dealing.

The developmental history of the *self-system* implies the circumstances under which the interviewee will experience anxiety—at least momentary anxiety—and sets the general patterns of the security operations which will be manifested

---

[1] [*Editors' note:* Sullivan says in his Notebook that this use of 'himself' is "a locution that is descriptive of phenomena rather than a precise statement."]

under these circumstances. The developmental history of the *person*, which includes the developmental history of the self-system, is accessible to the interviewer only in the form of: (1) experience formulated *in* the self-system—even if it is manifested only in the form of *precautionary operations against* the clear recall and unmistakable showing of the effects of certain formative experience; and (2) data which form an adequate basis for inference about experience—and *deficiencies* in experience—of universal developmental significance. In other words, in one's dealing with an interviewee one is provided with data which are fairly clearly related to the developmental history of the interviewee's self-system, which is *manifested* in his security operations, his precautions against anxiety; and these data form a reasonably good basis for *inference* as to his deficiencies in a good, basic experience for living. In the first group, the signs are clear if the interviewer can read them; the second is always a matter of inference. It is from these considerations that the here-indicated technique for interviewing has its origin; from them comes the necessity for the interview situation to have a probable utility to the interviewee, the definition of the interviewer-interviewee relationship, or the physician-patient relation, as that of an expert and a client, and the setting up of four phases of the interview situation.

From these considerations arises also the principle that the interviewer needs to have a good grasp on some *schematization* of the way people, under the most fortunate circumstances, come to be as capable and as human as they are. Among all the schemata that have been useful to me in developing psychiatric ideas and building certain psychiatric techniques, the most useful—other than the concept that man is a highly adaptive creature and that a useful approach to a study of him lies in the observation of his interpersonal relations—has been the conception of the stages of his developmental history. I have mentioned that the interviewer must always have in mind one really pertinent question about the patient: "Who is this person and how does he come to be here?" The generic answer is that a combination of his native endowments and personal experience has brought him to this pass. I have already described how the interviewer may get a rough idea of the answer to this question in the reconnaissance. But how does he go about filling the gaps which are left in the social, statistical data? What is the thread which keeps him more or less on his course through the detailed inquiry? The best thread, so far as I know, is the developmental history. I have found the following heuristic classification of personality development to be useful: infancy, childhood, the juvenile era, preadolescence, early adolescence, late adolescence, and adulthood. I shall presently consider these eras at some length.

In addition, there are two gross categories of developmental history which seem pertinent in arriving at some plan for organizing the data: The first is the relationship between the serial maturation of ability that characterizes the earlier years—the first twenty-six or twenty-seven years of the human being after birth—and the probable opportunities for experience which the person has had. One cannot have an experience that requires ability not yet manifested; on the other hand, the fact that one has matured an ability does not in any sense guarantee him an opportunity to have experience to which the ability is peculiarly fitted. Thus there is always the problem of the coincidence of the opportunities for experience with the maturation of the abilities to have those experiences. The second category, much more complex than the first, is made up of signs of personality warp uncovered in the interview. Such signs are evidence of deficiencies in needed experience—that is, needed in the sense that every one of us must have it to grow up—and are also indications of security operations pertaining to these deficiencies, which not only reflect the deficiencies but also limit or distort the recognition of, and the profitable utilization of, subsequent opportunities for remedying the deficiencies. In the last part of this statement I refer to one of the basic truths in the understanding of personality: as the self-system develops it shows a very potent tendency to influence, if not to control, the direction of its immediate future development; thus security operations actually stand in the way of the patient's gaining the experience that would remedy those deficiencies in earlier living which initially gave rise to the security operations.

According to my outline of personality development, the first stage, *infancy*, begins at birth and ends with the appearance of articulate speech, however uncommunicative. During this brief period, the expansion of human potentialities goes on at a truly prodigious rate. The learning of speech habits—or, in certain cases, the indication that speech habits could be learned—ushers in the era of *childhood*. In childhood the velocity of development, which has already begun to slow down at the end of infancy, continues to diminish. Nevertheless, those things that are learned in childhood—speech, toilet habits, and so on—are of such spectacular importance that it still seems as if the child learns with almost lightning speed. Even though mothers are sometimes not greatly impressed by this speed, anyone who tried to teach these things to an adult who knew none of them would realize that the child is incredibly educable, and is able to catch on to new things in a positively dumbfounding way.

During infancy and childhood, a "significant adult" has appeared as a queer kind of creature not clearly comprehended but of great importance as a source of the exceedingly uncomfortable experience of anxiety. But only at the end of childhood does each of us develop a need for the "other," in the sense of someone who is like us and is quite clearly *not* a significant adult. In other words, childhood ends when the child begins to show a need for compeers—a discriminating interest in, or rather realistic fantasies of, other playmates. Now there are some infants who have what adults may call "playmates," and certainly quite a number of children *seem* to have them. But the "play" in which these people are "mates" is actually composed of the independent operations of two entities, each of whom makes some minor accommodations to the presence of the other.

The need for compeers ushers in what I call the *juvenile era*. This stage is chiefly characterized in our culture by its relationship to school and formal education. Learning at this time continues at a somewhat diminishing rate, perhaps because of the increasing complexity of that which must be learned—"complexity," in my usual sense, meaning incongruity and lack of rational principle. Up to this time, the culture has been transmitted to the child by as few as two, three, four, or five people, and of necessity it has been distorted by their particular outlooks and peculiarities. But now many of the errors in the juvenile's acculturation which have existed because of the peculiar warp of his home are corrected by contact with other juveniles who also have ideas of what is right and proper, learned in *their* homes. All of these things tend to focus in minor respects on the teacher, and the formal education tends to show the juvenile what is unquestionably wrong, and what is unquestionably right, in what he knows already.

Another learning process which appears at this time can only be carried on with compeers, and not with significant older people: the juvenile discovers that he has certain successes and failures in competition—that is, in performances in which he falls into active comparison with another, more or less similar, person. And along with this, the juvenile learns that at times it is very necessary to compromise, and that there are certain ways in which he can compromise without loss of self-respect, and without being humiliated as a weakling. And as the years of schooling go on, the juvenile learns that he gets status for being bright, or for being teacher's pet, or for being popular, or for playing football, and things of that kind.

At the end of the juvenile era, another great developmental change appears. This may occur anywhere between the ages of eight and a half and ten, or even later, for the stages of development grow progressively less fixed in their relation to chronological age—a reflection of the influence of acculturation on maturation. The change which ends the juvenile era is rather startlingly abrupt—that is, it is a matter of weeks; however, this abruptness is apparently never noticed by the person who undergoes it. He begins to show positively adult caution in that he doesn't say very much about it until he gets used to it; as a result, his family has, at first, little awareness of the new occurrence. The change is this: One of those compeers of the same sex, who has been so useful in teaching the juvenile how to live among his fellows, begins to take on a peculiar importance. He is distinguished from others like him by the fact that his views, his needs, and his wishes seem to be really important: he begins to matter almost as much, or quite as much, as does the juvenile himself; and with this, the juvenile era ends and the phase of *preadolescence* begins. This person who becomes so important is ordinarily referred to as a *chum*, and he matters even when he isn't there, which is quite unlike anything that happened in the juvenile era.

During preadolescence, certain dramatic developments, which are probably necessary to elevate the person to really human estate, move forward with simply astounding speed. During this brief period, which may precede puberty by a matter of only weeks, or, more commonly, months, there is an acceleration of development, which, if one likes to think physiologically, may reflect the oncoming puberty change. Be that as it may, in the new-found importance of another person, there is a simply revolutionary change in the person's attitude toward the world. Thus far, regardless of his parents' fond belief in his utter devotion to them, and regardless of his ability to get along with his compeers, it is measurably correct to say that the young human has been extraordinarily self-centered. The startling change in preadolescence is that this egocentricity, this concentration on one's own satisfactions and securities and the wonderful techniques at one's disposal for obtaining them, now ceases to be the primary goal in living. The thing that seems most important now is the using of all these techniques to draw closer to another person. It is what matters to this other person, the chum, that is of the utmost importance. In other words, here is the first appearance of the need for intimacy—for living in great harmony with someone else. Because the need for intimacy makes the other fellow and living in harmony with him of such importance, a great deal of attention is paid to how he thinks and "feels," to what he likes and dislikes; and from this more careful observation of the other is gathered a great deal of data on the rest of the world. As long as

Little Willie was learning his geography, giving the right answers in school, and all that sort of thing, it might be inferred that he had a very intense interest in visiting Germany or Canada, or in learning the multiplication tables, although such interests didn't hound him in his sleep. When, however, he discovers that life cannot really be complete without an increasing closeness and harmony with someone else, he begins to develop quite rapidly a personal interest in the larger world.

I believe that the best grasp on the problems of life that some people ever manifest makes its appearance in these preadolescent two-groups. Such comprehension is often horribly unlettered and in woefully undocumented form, but it includes a remarkable awareness of another person and a quite astonishing ability to reveal oneself to that other. Because our culture is so forbidding to the development of certain human expressions, the next step in personality development is frequently accompanied by a state of being more or less chronically anxious—and the chronically anxious are not apt to have very free, constructive, and philanthropic interests in their fellow men. Thus the brief epoch of preadolescence very often represents the maximum achievement of a particular person, as far as a constructive interest in the welfare of the world is concerned.

The puberty change comes along at the end of preadolescence, and for a time the course of events does not seem to be greatly disturbed by changes in the voice, the appearance of new hair, and so on. The last astonishing physiological maturation of which we know is the appearance of the orgasm, by which I mean nothing more mystical than, in the male, the simple ejaculation of semen. Some time after ejaculation is established, he (to continue using the male as our example) begins to feel that one of the girls is far more attractive than he had previously noticed, and does something about his discovery. His chumship then disintegrates rather rapidly, and the youth wanders into *early adolescence*, in which, to be very crude about a magnificent and very troubled period, he attempts to find a pattern of life which includes the satisfactory discharge of lust. Even after he has found something in the way of a technique, so to speak, to deal with this drive which appears with the puberty change—and which, if unsatisfied, is apt to be extremely troublesome—he may spend several years more, if not the rest of his life, in attempting to learn how to get other people to collaborate with him in dealing with it.

When a pattern of life is achieved which satisfies this drive, *late adolescence* has begun. It continues until, through many educative and eductive steps, the person is able, at *adulthood*, to establish a fully human or mature repertory of interpersonal relations, as permitted by available opportunity, both personal and cultural.

These are the classical developmental eras of personality; for each of these I have given a threshold point which is very rich in its implications, and which must have profound significance for the future of the person. In each of these eras of personality development there are certain experiences which are the ordinary lot of the comparatively fortunate human being; and if—perhaps because of peculiarities of the parental group to which the person is subjected—these experiences cannot be had, they show, until they are remedied, as serious deficiencies in the development of personality, with many concomitant signs and some symptoms. And it is these deficiencies which make up the principal business of the psychiatrist, as well as the business of those concerned with the adjustment of personalities to jobs. Of course, there is unquestionably some difference in what an interviewer can investigate in interviewing a person for the position of fifteenth vice-president in charge of operations of a manufacturing company, compared to what a psychiatrist can do in interviewing a patient. But while there are differences in what the interviewer can ask and what attitude he can manifest, and so on, there are no differences in the significance of the data that he must seek to obtain.

A Suggested Outline for Obtaining Data

I wish now to give some hints as to the type of approach, type of surmise, which may be useful in conjunction with the developmental history in order to learn the important details about the interviewee and how he has come to be who he is. I trust you will realize that this is not a definitive outline—there are unnumbered things which do not appear in it; but from a consideration of your own recallable past, you will see that this outline hits the high points, and you can utilize your own past to fill in many of the details.

DISORDERS IN LEARNING TOILET HABITS

One of the first things which the interviewer might obtain information about is the patient's history of learning 'toilet habits.' The establishing of such patterns is usually begun before the end of infancy, and as a result the patient's information about them is probably not formulated and would require months of investigation to bring to any state of certainty. Thus almost no one knows consciously much about his own toilet training. But often he has picked up some clues about it.

Some of the really unfortunate people of the world have been exposed to strict bowel training well before early childhood, and as a result of their parents' preternatural interest in their toilet habits (which interest is but one expression of the parents' personalities) have come to suffer rather grave disturbances of life thenceforth. In other words, the very early learning of perfectionistic toilet habits—occurring well in advance of the appearance of speech, however autistic in nature—may lead a person to show very serious warp from the average course of human development from thenceforth, unless more fortunate experience occurs later.

The very driven, obsessional parent who teaches his children to be extremely tidy before they have any chance of developing those patterns of expression which should have gone on nicely before they became tidy, is usually so proud of the achievement that he brags of it every now and then to sort of puff himself up with how good he has been. A child usually learns of all this by hearsay from the parent to whom it was terribly significant that the child be wonderfully tidy from a very early age.

The patient, however, won't think of all that in a psychiatric

interview; and, even if asked directly, he may be so dashed by
the scope of the inquiry—if not by the apparent irrelevance of
it—that he may be intensely annoyed and quickly put an end
to it. So the interviewer looks for such little signs as he may
notice in this connection. Such signs are often obscure. I know
nothing which is peculiarly indicative of extremely early tidiness or very belated tidiness. But I do know that disorders of
toilet habits may be obscurely reflected—to the extent of a significant statistical coincidence—in personal cleanliness and in
certain other things. Among these are the attention given to the
dust which may have accumulated on chairs on which one is
about to sit, to the keeping of clothing from any casual contact
with dirt, to the careful preservation of creases in trousers, and
so on. Such things are hints which suggest that it might presently be worth while for the psychiatrist, without any undue
precipitateness, to make some inquiries as to the family mythol-
ogy about how early the patient became tidy. In my inquiry I
tend to emphasize the *estimable qualities of the abnormality*—
thinking that no one need feel great shame or offense at my
noting some particular neatness or carefulness in his dress. I do
not wish to frighten the interviewee away by too blunt reference to a carefulness that he might consider peculiarly private
or 'strange.' Parents who have produced tidy infants are usually
so proud of it that the child later hears about it; and so I come
to hear also.

This personal cleanliness pertains not only to whether the
patient is coarsely dirty, but also to how carefully he has
combed his hair, cleaned his fingernails, shaved, and all that sort
of thing. Fortunately, since we know so much more than we
usually get formulated—otherwise we would long since have
died from exhaustion—we can fairly easily get an impression
of whether a person is clean, is unkempt or unclean, is tidy,
or is positively neat. The feeling that a person is ordinarily
clean, and not unduly clean or unduly dirty, is the norm; that
condition indicates that the patient has no preternatural interest
in this field.

Disorders in learning toilet habits may also be reflected, more subtly, in the patient's attitude toward certain words, which he regards as definitely offensive and does not use. Such words are those which are ordinarily considered 'dirty' words by juveniles. Since they are not ordinarily used by psychiatric interviewers, it is a little bit difficult to get at this. But nonetheless the interviewer keeps such things in mind. A psychiatrist may gradually realize that a patient is a little restricted in his freedom to use such words as he knows. If, after the initial interview, the psychiatrist takes such a patient for intensive psychotherapy and gives him the old psychoanalytic prescription that he should lie on the couch and say every littlest thing that comes to his mind, he probably will sweat and blush, and one thing and another, for several hours, because the only thing that comes to his mind is one of these Anglo-Saxon words that he can't say. That is interesting, but it is also a poor technique for saving time.

Among the things that one may think of as related to the period of toilet training are prolonged enuresis (years past the time that most people cease to wet beds), habitual constipation, recurrent diarrhea (episodes of diarrhea so frequent that one never knows from week to week, or day to day, when the next one will come), and even an occasional soiling of the bed. Unthinking bluntness about matters such as these may only serve to block communication. It is helpful for the interviewer to have in mind the possible meaning of little hesitancies and so on. With such meanings in mind, he can find times at which he can ask, quite frankly and simply, and obviously for professional information, rather pointed and ordinarily prohibited questions. However, he can do this successfully only if he has caught on to the clues that make such questions relevant. If the interviewer asks a number of pointed questions that prove to be irrelevant, then he is not showing the skill in interpersonal relations which the client expects of him. But if he asks relevant questions at times when they are faintly apropos, the patient will probably not be at all offended and will be able to give relevant information.

DISORDERS IN LEARNING SPEECH HABITS

Since, in the more fortunate, the learning of speech habits usually collides with the learning of toilet habits, so that one or the other seems to be neglected for a little while, the interviewer next thinks, in the developmental scheme, of disorders in learning speech behavior. Such disorders may show up in faint suggestions of earlier trouble (such as hesitancy in speech), in oral overactivity, or in manneristic accompaniments of speech at times of stress.

If an interviewer is interested in such phenomena, he may notice that a patient shows a little tendency to hesitancy in speech at those times when he seems to be a little embarrassed about one thing or another. The second time this occurs, the interviewer can pause and, making a somewhat abrupt transition, say, "Tell me, did you stutter as a child?" And lo! he learns that the patient did. A great many people who have had serious speech disorders show some suggestion of an impediment in speech at times of stress for many years after they have overcome the more gross disorders. It is not so difficult to notice these signs, but there are others whose relationship to difficulties in speech development is not at first so easy to observe. There are some people, for example, who show, while talking, a good many obscurely unnecessary movements of the face around the mouth—which I call oral overactivity. There are others who display various mannerisms while talking; for example, a person may have to pause for a moment and do something, such as gesture with his hand, before he is able to speak freely.

All of these things suggest that there may be great value in developing an interest in the distortions of personality occurring as far back as the learning of speech. The signs that come to the interviewer's attention may all have some relationship to a history of disorders or deficiencies in speech habits, which the interviewer can discover by careful questioning. This history may show any of the following difficulties: (1) delay in learning to speak; (2) disturbed speech in the shape of stammering, stuttering, or lisping; (3) peculiarities of vocabulary; and (4) the continued use of autistic or frankly neologistic terms.

Delay in beginning to speak is not a disorder of learning speech behavior but a manifestation of a morbid situation in which there is no sufficient need for learning speech and, in fact, a positive premium on not learning. Lisping, which may be partly organic, has great social disadvantage and is therefore important to personality, however neurological or anatomical it may be in origin. The more obscure distortions, such as peculiarities in vocabulary, are not a disorder in acquiring speech behavior, but a defect in acquiring the knack of consensual validation—that is, the ability to move words around to the point that they convey what you mean to the person to whom you are going to speak.

Disorders in this last category are much more widespread than most people realize. As I have tried to suggest before, it is easy to believe that you understand everything said to you, and vice versa, but if you did not overlook negative instances, you would be greatly impressed with what queer things people mean by words that you use to mean something else. Sometimes the patient's use of words is extraordinary; he is apparently depending on a word to communicate something to you which it doesn't communicate at all, and you realize that he is still quite autistic in his verbal thinking and that there has been a very serious impairment of this extremely important aspect of his socialization. This reaches its positively pathological state in the use of neologisms which have meaning and existence as words only in the mind of the user. They are to be found in no dictionary, and they are not ordinarily subject to any of the philological laws. They are purely autistic, usually very highly meaningful, but utterly uncommunicative combinations of phonemes (that is, articulate sounds) which the person uses just as if they meant something to the hearer, and which cannot under any circumstances mean anything to the hearer except that they indicate the presence of a problem.

ATTITUDES TOWARD GAMES AND PARTNERS IN THEM

We now move into the juvenile era, admittedly leaving a great deal of an exceedingly rich period untouched, such as all the attitudes toward authority which have their buttresses in childhood, in the gradual domination of the parents over certain unregenerate impulses of the child, and so on. If you glance back into your school years, one of the things that may impress you immediately is that you were inducted into games which represented a certain cooperation, a certain element of competition, and often a very large element of compromise with compeers. That, I sometimes think, is the easiest approach to understanding the development of idiosyncrasies in the juvenile era. I hope that an interviewer will always get some idea of his client's attitude toward games and toward the people who are his partners in these games.

There are some wonderful eccentricities that appear here. A certain small section of Manhattan society rise from bed in the late forenoon, dress rather carefully, gather up their husbands or wives—their concessions to social necessity, as it were—and proceed to the bridge club. There they engage in an intensely concentrated performance, almost without speech or with only very highly formalized speech. After a considerable number of hours at this, they go out and retrieve their social remnant—by which I mean their mate—get something to eat, and go through a practically meaningless routine of life until the next meeting of the group. These utter devotees to bridge, thanks to the peculiarities of the Manhattan concentration of eccentricity and so on, do live a life which is all bridge; the rest is a matter so obviously of boring and tedious routine that it is very impressive. If you should feel very superior to these queer people, let me suggest that I don't find them to be very much different—except in the completeness with which they have organized their lives around what they want to do—from certain large prosperous communities which center more or less around a suburban country club. In those instances all of life which is not involved in golf and the club is treated as a boring routine that one must go through. One's husband or wife who does something for a living to facilitate this pleasant life is obviously an infrahuman creature and is treated more or less as such. Now, these are truly juvenile people, but they have found very satisfactory ways of life. The fact that a person has been so sadly distorted at a certain phase of development that he doesn't get anywhere near being an adult does not mean that he becomes horribly abnormal and passes the rest of his life in a mental hospital. Far from it! It doesn't even mean that he is likely to become a candidate for a psychiatric interview, except in wartime and at other times when his volition doesn't have so much to do with what he does.

In any case, the interviewer can learn a good deal from inquiring into people's attitudes toward games. People who have had very stressful juvenile eras very probably are not members of New York bridge circles, or suburban clubs, or things of that kind. They are likely, in fact, to have a quite restricted interest in games and a very sharply restricted interest in people with whom to play them, but that is another story.

ATTITUDES TOWARD COMPETITION AND COMPROMISE

As I have said, there are some topics which one approaches somewhat indirectly, not wishing to arouse great anxiety by too blunt an exploration of some 'dangerous' ground. But the patient's attitude toward competition is a thing about which one can ask directly, since competition enjoys, if not great social esteem, at least great tolerance. There is no particular harm in asking the person before you what his attitude toward competition is. He will always say something interesting, if only "What do you mean?" On the topic of competition such an answer is amazing. Maybe he is puzzled by what you mean by "attitude." You can then inquire what puzzles him. If you get anywhere on that, you ask, "Well, what do you think of compromise?"—that is, what does the patient think of people who compromise, would he easily compromise, would he *never* compromise, *what* would he compromise on, and so on.

As all this goes on, the interviewer observes whether the in-

terviewee is manifestly competitive in the interview situation—
has to know more about things than you do, has to beat you to
what you are driving at—or, on the other hand, whether he is
unduly conciliatory in an effort to give you the feeling that he
agrees with even your lightest utterance. Such things are quite
significant; they may be overlooked or misinterpreted unless
the interviewer follows some sort of scheme for organizing his
thoughts and his procedure.

AMBITION

Among the people who have been relatively, if not absolutely, arrested in the juvenile era—in other words, whose subsequent development of personality has been either rudimentary or very much delayed—are some who, from their competitive nature, you might say, develop an intense ambition. This
ambition is usually rather clearly revealed by some remarkable
successes. This is a culture very rewarding of competition, and
within it anybody who sets his whole personality, tooth and
nail, on a certain type of thing is apt to have experienced astonishing successes and failures. It is worth while to notice not
only how intensely ambitious a person may be, but also the
character of the goal which is the point of his ambition. The
interviewer will discover a few people who are intensely ambitious about one thing after another; ambition is a characteristic of them, and the particular goal they are seeking seems to
be purely a function of the situation they are in. There are many
other people, more significant because they are quite apt to hold
important positions in society, who have been pursuing a more
or less well-defined goal for years and years, doing everything
short of homicide to get to it.

INITIAL SCHOOLING

In addition to competition, compromise, games, and what
not, the juvenile era is also the period of correcting the over-
individualistic warp of acculturation which nearly everyone
brings to the school from the home. It is particularly important
to distinguish, therefore, in one's thought and perhaps in one's

questions, the initial schooling. I do not refer to the first day of school, which unhappily has been so exciting that most people retain nothing but a foggy memory of it, but rather to the general period of grammar school. In the first place, everybody has been there, and in the second place, it is there that one begins so rapidly to learn social techniques to cover one's 'real' feelings that what happens thereafter is often not very revealing. The psychiatrist wants to know in general anything that will give him a notion of the way the patient felt toward grammar school. Did he have a good time? Did he learn a lot? Did he like to learn the sort of things that were offered there? Does he have the impression that some teacher was wonderful to him? And so on. In some ways this is a reflection of the happiness or unhappiness that he may have brought to school from his home.

One thing may be noticed which has a bearing on events in the juvenile era: this is simply that some people have a curious lack of facility for using the Anglo-Saxon. While it is practically impossible to talk English without using words derived from Anglo-Saxon, to some people words of Greek or Latin derivation seem to be much more attractive, more welcome, and more frequently used than their equivalents from the Anglo-Saxon. I, being one of these people, can tell you that a person may use words derived from Latin and Greek because Latin and Greek roots have been mixed up in the development of science. I started a science education very young, and was enamored of the precise reference which science had conferred on these Greek and Latin roots. That, however, doesn't explain those instances in which the use of the Anglo-Saxon becomes practically vestigial wherever a good Latin- or Greek-derived word can be used instead. If a person grows up in the home of a Latin or Greek professor, it probably isn't strange. But it is of great interest when a person has grown up in a situation in which there was no obvious reason for distrust of the Anglo-Saxon, and in which it was the prevailing form of English used, and yet goes through life thereafter using chiefly words derived from Latin and Greek. It may be that he found in the accultura-

tion in school, and in the educational possibilities that opened
to him there, something much more attractive than anything he
had come to expect at home. And thus the interviewer may
gain, indirectly it is true, further knowledge of how the patient
felt about his home.

EXPERIENCE IN COLLEGE

If the interviewer's development of the inquiry too clearly
follows the developmental eras as I have set them up, he will, as
it were, be warning the interviewee of what 'should be' produced. In other words, he will be telling the interviewee what
security operations to use to defeat the purpose of the interview. Therefore, as I try to pick up the data from the very last
months of the juvenile era to maturity, topics are mentioned in
an order which I believe discourages a too easy appreciation of
just what is being driven at; yet this perhaps represents an exceedingly hurried sketch of what might, in the hands of the
skillful and the diligent, be an adequate outline of a prolonged
interview.

Rather abruptly, after asking something that is highly significant for the earlier years of the juvenile era, the interviewer can
leap over high school to college. Such sudden transitions disturb
the sets that are already beginning to develop in the patient, and
therefore improve the probability that he actually refers to his
recall instead of just attempting to adjust nicely to a certain
type of questioning. Thus, after having learned something
about the patient's experience in grammar school—for example, whether he was good in math or in English, or in both
(which is rare indeed)—I ask, if I have already learned in the
reconnaissance that he went to college, what was his experience
there. I ask if he fitted in with the "studes"—that is, the very
studious—or with the "socialites" at college. These are the two
groups into which most of the student body can be classified. So
far as one's future is concerned, under ordinary circumstances,
it is better to be one or the other than to be the exception. And
in America, unless one really has a career spreading before
one, it is better to be a social success than to be a stude. In other

words, the American pattern of normality is to go to college
and spend your parents' money, and to avoid any information
that you can elude; that is the more 'normal' pattern of development. Remember, norms are not given by God, or by you, but
are the outcome of statistical nose-counting. So, the interviewer
wants to know where his patient stood in college. Was he identified with the unduly studious, or the unduly frivolous, or was
he not identified?

INTEREST IN BOYS' OR GIRLS' CLUBS

The interviewer also inquires whether his patient, before he
became a father—or before she became a mother—showed any
particular interest in leading boys' or girls' clubs, in being a "big
brother" or a "big sister," for a period of years. If he did, I think
it is a fairly important clue to deficiencies in his preadolescent
experience.

THE PREADOLESCENT CHUM

Having reached this point in the interview, I usually inquire
whether the patient had a chum in the preadolescent era. The
preadolescent change has so much to do with one's social adap-
tability, one's actual place in at least the potential world of the
future, that not to have gotten some experience along this line
seems to me very unfortunate. Since there would seem to the
interviewee to be little direct connection between whether he
had an interest in boys' clubs and whether he had a chum, I like
to have a little transition. Without any great show of abruptness, I try to indicate that everything breaks here, and we are
starting on an entirely new line. Then I inquire, "Does anyone
stand out in your recollection as having been especially your
chum in your early school years?" If the answer is in the affirmative, I wish to learn what became of the friendship and of
the friend. Are they still great friends?

There is so much looseness in speech about these relationships that a categorical question such as mine is quite necessary
if, in the space of a minute or two, you are to get some useful
clue. You can be wonderfully misled in this field. Many people

think that they ought to have had chums, and they are glad to enumerate fifty or so that they did have. But when you say, "Does anyone stand out in your recollection?" the "anyone" means the chum is singular and indicates that the patient may have to say who, and what, and which, and why he was. Thus the patient usually pays a little serious attention to the question, rather than making an immediate social gesture to indicate his normality and so on. The further inquiry as to what became of the relationship gives the interviewer some notion as to its true character—whether it is an imaginary construct or an excerpt from life. Quite often the patient has not thought of his chum for twenty-two years, so that he is a little dashed by the question for a moment, but is able to say, "Yes, I had a chum, but I can't think of his name." If he is astonished that he can't think of the chum's name after twenty-two years of not using it, this is a strong confirmation of his having had one. Thus the outcome is often quite convincing, and after listening to what the patient has to say in response to a categorical stimulus like this, you feel pretty sure that you know what was the case; whereas any casual questions, or careless leading up to the subject, may bring conventional, obscuring responses that are likely to be quite far from the true facts.

PUBERTY

Then I often ask, "When did you undergo the puberty change?" I ask this merely to introduce a topic, because not one out of perhaps seventy or eighty people has the ghostliest idea of when he underwent the puberty change. The person was old enough to remember, but events then were so disconcerting, so much was going on at that time, that it's like the first day at school—everything is in a fog. I vividly remember the experience of one day trying to whistle and finding that I couldn't; but I haven't any idea as to what day or year it was. So it is with most people. But it doesn't do any harm now and then in the interview for the patient not to know the answer to something asked directly.

You then inquire about certain things: when the patient's voice changed, when he began to shave, and when he had orgasm; or in the case of a woman, when she first menstruated, when she noticed changes in the breasts, and so on. On all of these things most people are extremely vague. Yet, as you enumerate them, the patient may recall something important about one of them. If the patient's puberty was very late, which may be very significant, he is likely to recall something about more than one. That is really the most significant thing about the puberty change: if it occurs two or three years after most of the people in the patient's group have undergone it, this delay may be in itself a sign of very serious warp in personality, and in turn causes further increasing warp in personality. Under those circumstances, a great deal of the misery in life is dated to the actual delay in puberty change, and about all this the patient will have a remarkable amount of information. That in turn means a great deal about the misery of life that has separated that time from now.

Once I have gone through the process of being unable to determine at what age a patient became pubescent, I am able to inquire somewhat further about these phenomena, and I try to find out whether there were any unfortunate ideas connected with them. If I then learn that there are concrete recollections —for example, a woman may say something like, "I thought that something must have gone dreadfully wrong because I never dreamed of anyone bleeding there"—I know that there was indeed unfortunate experience. However, if I were to go about it the other way and say to the woman, "Did your mother warn you about it?" or "Did you know what was going to happen?" she could only reply, "Of course Mother did" or "Of course Mother didn't." And with such answers I wouldn't know anything. First I verify the fact that the interviewee does or does not know when puberty happened, but at least knows what I am talking about, and then I learn if there were any unfortunate ideas connected with the event. With this indirect approach I may come to know something which is reasonably trustworthy.

UNFORTUNATE RELATIONSHIPS IN EARLY ADOLESCENCE

Having gone thoroughly over all the amnesias, and so on, of the puberty change, I then ask, again rather categorically, "Is anyone recalled as having been a particularly bad influence in early adolescence?" Should the patient after a moment's thought say "Yes," I use my judgment of the degree of his anxiety as to whether to proceed any further on that topic. If the answer is in the affirmative, I more generally leave the matter right there rather than inquire into it, but I try not to forget it since such data may be developed later. It is very seldom important to know all about this unfortunate relationship. The important thing is that there does seem to have been such a relationship, and in many, many instances it is well to restrain your curiosity and to confine yourself to the significant question of what became of that relationship. If it has been treasured ever since, that's interesting; if, on the other hand, it was exterminated as soon as possible, that sounds pretty healthy.

ATTITUDE TOWARD RISQUÉ TALK

The interviewer then asks about the patient's recollections of the pornographic art in the school conveniences, his memories of the types of obscenities heard in high school, and so on, and how the patient felt about them. If he is comparatively well, the patient, very vaguely and without any conviction, guesses that he didn't like them at first, which is correct. The interviewer then moves very suddenly into the present and wants to know what the patient thinks of risqué or frankly sexual talk. Does he participate in it easily? Does he find it rather repellent? And so on. If the patient seems to you to be quite eccentric, and you are still terribly at sea, you might ask him if he feels that such sexual talk is obscene. Now, what "obscene" means to one person is probably different from what it means to another, but in this culture, "obscene" usually carries a very vigorous condemnation. Thus it is not unusual for a person to be embarrassed by risqué stories. However, when a person feels that all risqué stories are positively obscene—when they would not impress most people as such—he has probably been subjected to pretty warping influences in bygone years and hasn't escaped from them.

ATTITUDE TOWARD THE BODY

Having gotten some hints as to the freedom with which the patient can contemplate the fact that he or she has genitals, without ever having mentioned them, you may then take up a somewhat related topic: namely, does the patient's attitude toward his genitals apply also to the rest of his body? A gentle way to approach this, if you have learned nothing from the discussion of games and sports, is to ask if the patient is a member of the YMCA, an athletic club, or something of that kind, and to ask what he does in such a place. If the patient turns out to be a member of the swimming team, for example, the chances are that he is willing to have some of his skin seen in public, and you don't need to ask foolish questions about that.

If you have led up to it so that he doesn't think you have an unjustifiable curiosity of some kind, you ask him if he has any remaining objection to being seen nude by people of the same sex. If he hasn't, then you can ask him if he still feels a little modest about some parts of his body. This can be interesting. In other words, you are trying to pick up some idea of the patient's attitude toward his genitals and the rest of his body.

SEX PREFERENCE

Having led the patient to thinking a little in terms of later adolescence, you can ask whether he actually prefers men or women for companionship. If the patient shows a little increase in reserve at this point, you can always modify your question amiably by saying, "Well, it may vary with the moods that you're in. Of course you would prefer the company of women when you are retiring with a view to sexual satisfaction." If he looks suspiciously at you, you were wrong—which is information. And you can continue by asking the patient whom he likes to dine with, and so on.

Now, the preference for members of the other sex really

does vary from situation to situation in most people. And yet the interviewer's general questioning should proceed in the fashion I have outlined. You can't be too precise in questions without getting the patient somewhat startled. In other words, you ask general questions fairly often merely as a method of transition, to get a topic into the open. Having accomplished this, you become specific.

ATTITUDE TOWARD SOLITUDE

The interviewer should also find out what his patient's attitude toward solitude is. There are, believe it or not, some people who regard the possibility of solitude as the better among you regard your reward in heaven—except that they find their reward now. There are other people who would really run four miles to avoid solitude. And there are many in between. If the patient either likes solitude or doesn't seem to know what it means—in other words, probably doesn't need it very often—then the interviewer can ask this rather categorical question: "Are you ever so lonely that you become restless?" (Now, this is not "Were you ever" or "Do you recall," but "*Are* you ever.") The answer is highly significant when it is in the affirmative.

USE OF ALCOHOL AND NARCOTICS

By all these techniques, I have covered the developmental history except for neglecting attitudes toward authority which I shall not attempt to cover here. And now I come to a few other topics which seem to me to require very special consideration. They are not at all as rewarding, or as basically significant, as is the notion of the developmental history, but they serve their purpose.

The first that I will mention is the relationship of the interviewee to alcohol or narcotics. A good many psychiatrists overlook the possibility of the use of narcotics, which is of course very much more restricted as an outstanding idiosyncrasy than is the use of alcohol. But don't utterly forget narcotics, because you do sometimes see a drug addict.

This business of alcoholic beverage is something which I think is revealing enough so that I seldom fail to inquire about it. I shall run very swiftly over some of the things I like to find out. When was the patient first drunk? I say "drunk" with a slight falling inflection to apologize for the idea that he could ever have been drunk. The patient usually tells me. Nearly everybody has been drunk for a first time. The really interesting thing is whether he got drunk again. After the patient has survived the shock of my thinking that he may have been drunk, I ask him if he has ever been fairly seriously injured when under the influence of alcohol, or more or less because he was intoxicated. It is remarkable what a large proportion of people have been deterred from going down the alcoholic road by suffering some rather serious injury when they were drunk, or an accident that might have had serious consequences; such people have gained certain high discretion about the blending of alcohol with dangerous activities. So it is worth knowing about that.

Then I wish to know what the patient does when he takes quite a bit of liquor. Does he become quarrelsome? Does he engage in fights? Does he develop crying spells or weep easily? Or does he become very friendly with everyone? The answer very frequently is, "I get sleepy"—which is not always true. In those cases in which the patient indicates that he shows a very disagreeable complex of behavior when drunk, but is not eager to talk about it, I don't question further. Such behavior indicates a very unhappy person who takes to alcohol when social pressure is too high and who, under the loss of inhibitions, reveals a good deal of the misery and hostility which have led him into grief with society. Quarreling and pugnacity are more or less degrees of the same thing, and are, so far as I am concerned, definitely suggestions that the personality is not excellently integrated, and has not achieved a high degree of development in late adolescence.

I then ask the patient how much he can "carry"—that is, how much alcohol can he ordinarily take with no serious inconvenience to coordination or judgment. When he has given me some kind of answer—usually rather vague, because here again I am introducing a topic more than expecting data—I want to know what circumstances provoke him to exceed this amount. I sometimes hear amazingly revealing things. In other words, many people are so distressed at their incapacity at times to avoid excessive alcohol that they have actually worked out a pretty good pattern of the situations that provoke them to do so. I then wonder if the patient has noticed anything which alters his capacity or tolerance for liquor. There are a good many people who can drink a great deal most of the time, but who at times become intoxicated on a remarkably small amount. If the patient has noted something like that, he may also have been so impressed by the risk connected with it that he has actually figured out some data on what seems to affect him.

Having gotten all this, I may ask something to determine to what extent the person is a connoisseur—that is, how insistent he is on either the variety or the quality of alcoholic beverage. There are people who, other things being unobtainable, take ethyl alcohol, with or without water; there are other people who are so unpleasant about not having what they want that their intimate friends always see that the right kind of liquor is available before having them in. That is not merely a peculiarity of the drinking habit; it is also a reflection of one's importance, both to oneself and to others, and is, from that point of view, rather interesting. People who have nothing to go on in the way of self-respect are not apt to be connoisseurs.

I then want to know just how emphatic are these matters of taste? If I find out that they are quite emphatic, I wish to learn how this great emphasis is explained or rationalized. I don't really care about the rationalization; I simply want to hear the patient talk about this emphasis on taste. His comments will give me a clue as to how seriously he takes himself, what he may have learned from experience, and many other things which appear in the rationalizing of any strong taste or insistent preference.

EATING HABITS

Next, I may inquire about matters of eating. There is no personal preference shown in my putting alcohol before eating. Alcohol is actually a much better introduction to a whole state of mind than eating would be, since everyone eats, and usually not entirely to his satisfaction. I almost always, even at Army induction centers, want to know about the state of the stomach and bowels, and I ask, "Does any food disagree with you?" And, of course, in a twenty-five-dollar-an-hour practice one asks, "Are there any food allergies?" This makes a most respectable introduction to the general topic of eating. I then ask, if I haven't been told, if there is any food that the patient dislikes—in other words, is he notional about food. If he is, this, in general, reflects a considerable interest, even if a highly pathological one, in food matters in very early years. Sometimes I hear a history to the effect that the patient once disliked this and that, but that the Army cured him of it. Such an account is interesting, because that is a type of stress that many people have never undergone. I want to know if the patient is a heavy or light eater, if he has irregular meals, if he eats late at night, and so on. Sometimes such things are quite interesting to learn —and often they seem to be drearily irrelevant. You must use some judgment as you go along.

In case of an unusual, puzzling, or quite possibly very important person, it is well to get at the question of how ceremonially he treats the meals for which he has time. Now, oddly enough, some extremely busy people have time for lunch. They enjoy the ceremony of lunching with certain people, whereas to eat dinner at home may be dully routine. Is some particular meal likely to be treated rather ceremonially? In other words, does the patient give a considerable amount of attention to arrangements, to things being right, and does he experience considerable distress if, for example, the Blue Points run out at the restaurant and he can't have what he expects? All this is an interesting reflection of the patient's attitude toward life. Even his attitude toward friends may come out in this consideration of the extent to which some meal comes to be a real occasion which he looks forward to and takes a good deal of interest in and trouble about.

SLEEP AND SLEEP FUNCTIONS

The interviewer next hints at the sleep habit and the sleep functions. If he does not lead up to this topic with some careful inquiry, he will often draw only misleading blanks. Sleep functions are known to most people only by way of their dreams. But if you think of the phenomena as *sleep* and the *sleep functions*, you will be a little safer than if you thought, in the traditional way, of just sleep.

One way to introduce this topic is to ask, "How much sleep do you seem to need?" If the patient tells you, well and good; if he doesn't, you are at least in the field and can ask further questions, such as whether he is a heavy or light sleeper, whether he sleeps well in strange beds or Pullman berths, and so on. You then ask if he ever dreams. Some people will consider that question just too naïve for words, and others will say "No" with perfect honesty, as far as they know. If the patient dreams, you ask whether he ever has nightmares. Sometimes you come upon a curious phenomenon—the person who doesn't dream but who has nightmares. I tell you, you don't know what people mean, or what your words mean to them, until you find out!

In some cases, where everything seems to be most shockingly normal, I may indicate that I am not too pleased to discover that the patient sleeps eight hours every night, never dreams, and never had a nightmare. Looking at the poor patient somewhat irritably, I say, "Did you ever have night terrors? Did anybody tell you about your having night terrors?" I suppose about half the human race doesn't know what night terrors are, but if you have had them, you do know. The recollection is usually sufficiently unpleasant that the patient gives a sign of it, no matter what he wishes to conceal. If he has had night terrors and has been a little discomposed by my irritation and my question, I ask again what he dreams when he does dream—this last, in spite of his having told me that he never dreams. The patient may start to say again, "But I don't dream!" And I say, "Oh, I mean—recall a dream. Everybody has at least two or three dreams that he can remember, and I think that would apply even to you. What do you recall having dreamed ten, twenty years ago? Tell me a little something about your dream life." If he still has no dreams, I give it up as a bad job, figuring that here I am meeting a type of resistance that indicates one of two things: either the person has a very rigid self-organization, or he is a very guarded person who, under any pressure that I feel I can apply, still maintains what is obviously a very risky attempt to carry out his plan of being 'normal.' There are people who do not know they dream. Those people have a self-organization that, under sufficiently unhappy circumstances, would probably put them in a mental hospital, but would otherwise make them pillars of the church or of almost anything else that was highly respectable with which they happened to be identified.

THE SEX LIFE

Then we come to the topic of sex. You notice that I am quite interested in people's attitudes toward their genitals and in the history of certain changes which, at least in many people's minds, tend to concentrate in the genitals. I am not prodigiously interested in what can be learned in the early phases of a psychiatric interview by questions on sex. I particularly want to emphasize that the general doctrine that sex is in some curious fashion a mirror of personality is, so far as I can discover, capable of being astoundingly wrong. Sex is important for the twenty minutes it may occupy from time to time, but it is not necessarily behind everything else that fills the rest of the time.

If an interviewer has stumbled through all these topics in somewhat the fashion which I have suggested, he can say to the patient, "Well, and what of the sex life? Are you very restrained in such things, or are you quite free? Are you promiscuous?" That happy thought at the end sometimes gets big returns. Having gotten some kind of a sputter in response to that question, I ask, "Well, how long has it been true? I don't suppose you've always been like that. Give me a notion of the history of your sexual experience. For example, when did it begin?" When you know something about the beginning of the patient's developmental history, you may know what is being discussed; but missing the beginning, you often just *think* you know what is being discussed.

Some people, in fact a remarkable number of people, recall their first sexual encounter with another person; while it may be a little hard to place in time, it is usually vividly registered some way or other. If the patient tells me a little bit of something, I am satisfied. I don't care if it is not detailed at this time, because I have gathered almost all the data I need to guess about his great problems and his probable adjustment to the set of circumstances that may be before him. I am really sparring around for something I may have missed in everything that has gone before, and am not really looking for anything more intimately sexual than how he deals with members of the opposite sex—as friends or enemies. For example, if the patient is a man, is a large number of female conquests terribly important to his prestige? Or does he avoid intimacies with women, except for a dear old friend with whom he's been having them for twenty years? All of these things have much less to do with sex, you see, than they have to do with personality as a whole.

Having led the patient to think in terms of the backward glance, I then ask him something like (with women I may use something more by way of transition): "Was there much trouble over masturbation?" God pity us! I suppose that about three quarters of the people of my age immediately bridle and go through the motions of being terribly annoyed at the idea they ever masturbated. At these I look with a fine imitation of scorn, and say, "Now please don't tell me you never did. I don't believe I could stand that at my age. But now tell me, is there still some difficulty about it?" When that question is asked of people who have been married for eighteen years and have two or three children, they usually look at me sharply to decide whether to be indignant or not, but since it is just a question, they sometimes say "Yes."

Having given this awful shock, I may ask if the patient ever had any contact with prostitutes or streetwalkers. After listening to something or other on that topic I ask him if he has had venereal disease, and how often. I want to know if prostitutes are still of some considerable interest, and so on. Curiously enough, it has become increasingly apparent to me that in questioning either old men or young adolescents about their genital behavior, the same inquiries are relevant.

In certain cases I ask if the patient has had any experience with adultery. I don't ask that when I think it would be regarded as preposterous, but if I surmise that adultery is still a terrifying word to a person, I ask if he has engaged in it, how it affected him, and so on. In cases in which adultery wouldn't be of any interest to the patient or would seem a preposterous, archaic inquiry, I wonder if he has ever been involved, or threatened with involvement, in any divorce actions.

In case my informant appears to be notoriously normal—that is, vigorously but restrainedly heterosexual—I attempt by inquiry to discover whether his heterosexual genital performances are actually autoerotic in character—that is, using the genitals of the other sex in lieu of one's hands. I also attempt to discover whether his heterosexual performances are in the nature of a security operation—in which I wish to know how his having heterosexual relations contributes to his prestige, and so on. Last, I want to learn whether the patient's heterosexual genital operations are calculated to satisfy him and his partner.

COURTSHIPS AND MARRIAGE

That is a very reasonable sort of point at which to pass to marriage and the history of courtships, plural. If the plural doesn't apply, that in itself is interesting data. If you have developed the interview somewhat after the fashion that I have previously suggested, you are already warned from the social reconnaissance of a good many things with respect to marriage, courtship, children, and so on, pertaining to your interviewee.

Therefore you do not at an exceedingly late moment need to become curious as to whether the patient has consolidated the exceedingly important status performance of becoming a husband and father, or a wife and mother. That is one of the reasons for the reconnaissance. You gather all these overwhelmingly important data so that in the detailed inquiry you can proceed methodically without so much attention to the prestige necessities of the patient. In other words, the reconnaissance tells you what you will have to deal with when the proper time presents itself later in the detailed inquiry.

Next may come an assessment of interpersonal patterns, again plural, characterizing the married life—the satisfactions and dissatisfactions, and the securities and insecurities. When I use these alternatives, I refer to *every* case. I have yet to find a marriage which has only satisfactions and only securities. In other words, there may be many more satisfactions than dissatisfactions; but if a person tells me that his home life is perfect, I take off my glasses, which means I can't see him, and gaze at him, and say, "Extraordinary!" I then pass on to some other topic, but I return to this later.

I wish to know whether the mate is the person who runs things or the person who is run, or whether husband and wife happily share in their dominance over each other. And by whom outside of the marriage is the mate influenced: in-laws and so on, and particularly and never to be forgotten, the neighbors—in other words, to what extent is the mate harassed by a necessity of keeping up with the Joneses? Also, is there a sense of deep disappointment associated with the marriage relationship? Much of this you infer by the way the interviewee answers, not by asking him.

PARENTHOOD

Then we come to the mighty topic, if suitable, of parenthood. I try to assess the actual characteristics of the person as a parent, as well as his ideals of what he *should be* as a parent. And to those ends I ask such things as the awkward question: "Is there a problem child in the family?" If there is, what is the explanation considered to be? I also ask if there is a preferred child, and why that child is preferred. Has the preference had any bad effects on that child, or on any other child? If it has, are there any neutralizing influences that can be learned of from the informant? The attitude of the parent-interviewee to the school influences that are bearing on his child or children is an excellent entering wedge here, because school is somewhat impersonal. Then you want to know of grandparents, uncles, aunts, neighbors, and others who may be influencing his child or children.

There are two things to inquire about here which should not be forgotten. If you have been clever in your reconnaissance, you may already have some of these data. First, don't fail in the exploration of this area to discover if the wife has had any miscarriages and if some younger siblings died before the birth of the surviving child. In other words, you should know if such influences existed which would act to increase the importance of the surviving child, and so on. Second, inquire not only about half siblings, because there may have been a divorce on one side or the other, but also about wards or other pseudo-siblings in the family, people of approximately the same age who are looked after because for some reason there is not adequate care elsewhere. It is simply incredible how few hints you get of these things when they are significant, unless you ask about them.

VOCATIONAL HISTORY

After you get through all of these topics, you come to the vocational history. Remember that vocation in this culture usually means work, not esteem. Here again your reconnaissance in the second phase of the interview may have given you some excellent clues as to the advisability of working back with the person from his present vocation to get the history, or of starting at the very beginning of his vocational life.[2] If you decide

[2] [Editors' note: In a question-and-answer session at the end of the 1944 series of lectures, Sullivan was asked whether the patient's attitude toward his present job was of more significance than his attitude toward previous

to begin at the beginning, remember that in many homes some work contribution is required of the child long before he would be regarded as in any sense a wage earner. He may have had chores to do, and you want to know to what extent he did them, what compulsion he was under, and so on. You want to know about the first paid employment, about the first full-time employment, about any full-time vacation employment, and so

jobs. Sullivan discussed this point as follows, relating it to the investigation of current events in the patient's life:

"The attitude of a person toward the job that he's now working on is likely to be his attitude toward employment in general. What he reports about his attitude toward former jobs may consist of little more than the beautiful tinting effect of distance on memory. Thus I would certainly always want to know a good deal about a person's attitude toward his present job. If he says he is all for it, that is interesting; and I may find out whether that really is his attitude by inquiring whether he ever had any work that he didn't particularly care for. If he says that he doesn't like his present employment, I try to find out whether this has been his general attitude toward employment, or whether there are particular circumstances surrounding his present employment which justify considerable antagonism toward the situation.

"In general, in the treatment of personality there are three fields of events which are of very great relevance. The first of these is the field of current events in the patient's life outside the treatment situation—including his current employment. The second is his current relations in the treatment situation—that is, his relations with the psychiatrist. And the third field of relevant data is the events of the patient's past.

"It is difficult for most people to be straightforward and forthright in discussing their feelings, thoughts, impulses, and so on, with respect to a person with whom they are in the peculiar relationship of patient to psychiatrist. For a fairly long time at the start of all therapeutic work, therefore, most of our field of investigation is concerned with current events outside the treatment situation. One might not think so from reading some of the popularizations of psychoanalytic history, but this is nonetheless true. It is from current events that we move into the current therapeutic relationship between doctor and patient, uncovering both the noted and unnoted emotional problems which constitute the patient's difficulties in living.

"When we locate a problem, identifying something that is impractical, inefficient, and definitely contrary to the achievement of the patient's idealized goals, we have every reason to turn to the third field of greatly relevant data—the distant past in which this particular emotional difficulty had its beginning. It is important to notice that finding out how things start often provides a great deal of information as to what they represent, whereas their more sophisticated, mature manifestations may be very obscure indeed. However, some patients, as I have already said, have a distinct tendency to alter history to suit their wishes or needs; with them, the present has the virtue of being capable of at least some investigation, whereas the past is apt to be pretty heavily colored. From this general standpoint, what is currently going on has a very special significance."]

on. What happened to the earnings? What good did they do the person? Who used the earnings, and for what? Did they just get dissipated by the family, or were they used to buy roller skates or some other valuable thing? What training in thrift and all that sort of thing was received?

Note that in all occupational history you are actually attempting to learn about data pertaining to a job which is defined. It is simply incredible how wrong you can be if you merely assume that what a person says about his earlier jobs means what you think the words do. You attempt to discover what the interviewee did, his reasons for taking a job, his attitudes toward it, his retrospective idea of success or failure in it, and his status movement in taking it—that is, whether he dropped down or moved up in taking this job. Was the next job an upward move or a downward one? What is his retrospective attitude toward the skill-learning value of a particular job? Some people have hated some of their earlier jobs, but have thanked God for many years that they went through them because these jobs were helpful in skill-learning for some later occupation. As the interviewee looks back at it, was he encouraged or discouraged by his experiences in a job? Did the work in the job under discussion seem to have social usefulness? This is a very tricky thing because there are two approaches covered by the term "social usefulness": First, it refers to the effect of the job on the interviewee's self-respect. Self-respect is what important members of society reflect to you, so a job may improve your self-respect, or otherwise. Second, social usefulness may refer to the making of social contacts that have been useful subsequently. In other words, what was the outcome of the job with regard to the people the interviewee knew?

If you can keep track of all these criteria, you will know a great deal about a person just from investigating his vocational history.

AVOCATIONAL INTERESTS

The next thing to investigate is the avocational and recreational history. This is a very important field of data for the assessment of personality with respect to the degree of maturity of the person with whom you are dealing. Do not overlook the application of vocational criteria to avocational activities. Again, don't believe that because something sounds familiar to you, you know exactly what a person is talking about. When I finally developed the idea that I should ask two or three additional questions to find out what a person was talking about, I discovered, for instance, that the game of bowling actually means quite different things to different people.

The interviewer wants to know what is being discussed, you see, and he must take reasonable care to be sure that he knows what the thing really means to the person who is talking. This is especially important in dealing with the thoroughly immature, because their real interests in life are in their avocations, not in their vocations. Of such people you learn nothing much from the vocational history, but in a study of their avocational history you may discover something that begins to make sense. Even the most diligent people are more free in this field of avocation than the economic system permits them to be in vocational work. With this in mind, I have taken the trouble of trying to throw together a few hints of the field covered by avocational interests.

Every field of interest in avocational or recreational work has not only its own value, but also an importance as an area of contact with others. This contact with others, ranging from close to very remote, may be sharply restricted to the field of avocational interest or may show no restrictions whatever. Therefore, quite aside from the actual name of the avocation, there are always the problems of the relationship to the other people who participate in it.

There are, of course, a variety of fields of interest: the religious, the political, the social, and the scientific. It is of some importance in the organization of data about personality to distinguish among the various scientific fields—the social sciences, biological sciences, medical sciences, and human sciences.

Beyond the religious, political, social, and scientific is the aesthetic. When you come to that, look for the *fields*, because there are often more than one although one is conventionally presented. In all of these several aesthetic fields, you want to know whether the interest is manifested in passive or in active relationship. For example, does the interviewee spend hours looking at great oil paintings, or does he putter diligently making oil paintings? And in any aesthetic avocational interest, you want to know what the degree of socialization is. Is the interest something that the interviewee must share with other people who are doing it or is it something that he can do only if there is an appreciative audience that is not doing it?

Other avocational fields include the mathematical field of interest, the linguistic field, and the literary. This last divides sharply into the productive, the critical, and the consumptive. For those who read, what is the history of the books they like? Has their taste changed; or are they still devoted to detective stories as they have been since they can remember, or to mythologies as they have been for still longer; or have they gradually evolved a great interest in the classics and biographies?

The next great field of avocational interest is current history. Much more restful for some people is noncurrent history: the Civil War, medieval history, the history of pre-Hellenic culture, and so on.

In all these fields of interest there are important discriminations to be made among special aspects of larger fields. And we can learn much from the interviewee's particular avocational preoccupations, his reasons for developing these, the benefits or harm derived from them, and the role played by them in his relationships with other people. As we explore these interests, we learn to what extent the interviewee is aware of his fellow men, and of his own relationship to them and to their productions.

All of these things that I have touched on represent stresses, indices of direction of development, strong hints of persistent durable warp, and so on. Those are what we wish to learn about in the psychiatric interview. We are trying to find out who and what the person is. To do that we need to discover how he got where he is—and by what route he arrived. And the developmental history serves as a useful guide.

The Personified Self

I now wish to comment rather briefly on data to be obtained about the personified self, as contrasted with the personality as a whole. That about oneself of which one is from time to time clearly aware—that is, what one knows about oneself—makes up the data comprising the personified self. This is not the same as the self-system, for the personified self is necessarily less inclusive than is the self-system. The personified self is that "part," to use a locution, of the self-system which is reflected in statements pertaining to the subject, "I," and as such it is a source of communicated information, as contrasted with other information about the person's self-system which must necessarily be inferred. In other words, there is something of a distinction between what an informant can tell an interviewer, in contrast with what the interviewer can safely infer, and may, in fact, be able to validate by experiment, but about which the informant cannot tell him. What the informant can tell about his self-system is the content of the personified self.

I would now like to suggest a schematization of the personified self which is useful to the interviewer in this phase of the investigation:

(1) *What does the interviewee esteem and what does he disparage about himself?* It is a rare person indeed who disparages nothing about himself, but if he comes anywhere near wisdom, he is very chary about revealing what he disparages. It is, therefore, much easier to discover what a person really esteems about himself than it is to discover what he disparages. In the "perfect" psychiatric interview the interviewer discovers both what the patient esteems and what he disparages about himself.

(2) *To what experiences is the patient's self-esteem particularly, unreasonably, vulnerable?* In other words, what sort of situation puts him at an acute disadvantage against all of his reason?

(3) *What are the characteristic "righting movements"—security operations—which appear after the patient has been discomposed—made "consciously" anxious?* At this point I wish to draw attention to the distinction between these characteristic security operations at the times when the person knows that he has been made anxious, and those data which indicate the presence of security operations when the person does not notice that he has become anxious. I have already suggested that people often become annoyed, or irritated, or even angry when they have been made anxious, and never know that they have been anxious. The emotional state, the anger or hostility, has appeared so swiftly that the person is spared the realization that he has been anxious. But now I am talking about the security operations which appear in a different situation: the way that the person acts when he *knows* that he has been discomposed.

(4) *How great are the interviewee's reserves of security?* For instance: (a) *How well is the person's life justified?* How adequately, in other words, can the person state characteristics of his life which are, beyond reasonable doubt, estimable and worth while? (b) *Are there exalted purposes in his life which are demonstrated in action other than mere speech?* Speech is one form of activity in interpersonal relations. But for exalted purposes to be significant in validating the person's living and giving him a reserve of security, speech is not enough; he must have demonstrated those purposes in something other than mere statements. Speech may be terribly important in validating his living, but only if it is rigidly oriented toward a remote goal and not to the service of mere security operations. Thus the interviewer seeks to determine whether there are exalted purposes which the person has demonstrated over the years by something other than talk. (c) *Are there secret sources of shame or enduring regret?* And, if there are, what is their relation to the person's justification of his life? Those who are really in touch with what happens to them from the cradle to the grave almost always have some enduring regrets, and they are fortunate indeed if they escape durable shame about this or that. But that does not mean that such people lack a reserve of security.

Whether they have a great reserve of security depends on whether the justification of their lives as it exists in the personified self greatly outweighs their secret recriminations, shames, and regrets.

So far, I have named the four great criteria of the quality of the personified self that have proven durably useful in my experience. There may be many other criteria that would be better, but I have come to depend upon these. Now let me suggest some of the ways by which the interviewer discovers these things. In other words, I have tried to indicate what the interviewer wants to know; now I shall suggest *fields of data* which will shed some light on these major points.

Does the patient habitually seek to be regarded in a particular light? Does he seek to give the impression to most people that he is amiable, considerate, kind, and thoughtful; or—somewhat the reverse of these—does he seek to convey the impression that he is thoughtless, severe, cruel, inconsiderate, or austere? And remember that I am talking now about what the person *knows* that he seeks to convey. There are a notable number of people who go to a great deal of trouble to impress their environment with their austerity. These people may be among the most valuable citizens in the world, deeply and carefully considerate, very wise in their attempts at being kind. But I am talking about the impression on others that a person seems to be trying to convey; and that impression may vary from amiable to austere, from considerate to inconsiderate, from kind to severe or cruel, and from thoughtful to thoughtless. This merely indicates the way of showing himself to others which the person has consciously organized. It is significant as such, as the way he has found suitable for dealing with most life situations, and not as a product of the interview situation. And remember in this connection that I am discussing the data which arise from the standpoint of the accessible, or personified, aspects of the interviewee's self-system.

In this same inquiry, the interviewer wants to know what is the usual attitude manifested by the patient toward servants, and after some considerable digression, what attitude he manifests toward animals, meaning inferior creatures, domesticated or otherwise.

The interviewer may also usefully find out what are the characteristics of the person's attitude toward others in relatively unaccustomed contacts. That is, how does his attitude in *unaccustomed* contacts with certain groups differ from his attitude in *accustomed* contacts with them? Among such groups, I might name, first, those definitely superior, more fortunate, or wealthier. Second, I would mention people belonging to a different culture complex, such as those he encounters in a foreign country. A disturbance of attitude is particularly noticeable when the person is visiting in a country where there is a very considerable language barrier. In other words, this criterion of the personified self is more apparent in an American when he is on the Continent than when he is in England, for the English may seem quite natural to him, and even if they seem somewhat "odd," at least he can discuss their oddity with them. But when an American goes, for example, to France, Germany, Sweden, Spain, Italy, or Eastern Europe, then the element of foreignness is far more conspicuous to him, and the manifestations of his personified self become more striking. Also of interest are the characteristic attitudes in unaccustomed contacts with the definitely inferior, the less fortunate, or the less well-to-do.

It is important to note that the data that may be obtained pertaining to the *relatively unaccustomed* contacts may be quite different from those which are displayed in *recurrent* or *habitual* situations. A person may, in the course of making his living, have some contact with others who are definitely superior, more fortunate, wealthier, or more powerful, who fall in the general category of "bosses." He may be accustomed to participating in conference situations with people of much greater gifts than his own, to dealing with wealthy clients or with very poor clients, or to meeting those extraordinary people to whom one is likely to be introduced at cocktail parties. There are also many people, particularly those engaged in social work, who deal with clients whose background is, in a measurable sense, foreign to their own. And we all have certain contacts with people who are definitely inferior, less fortunate, and less well-to-do than we are. But such situations, if they are recurrent or habitual, are definitely less significant in the data they yield about the personified self than are parallel situations to which the person is really unaccustomed.

In addition to these things, the interviewer always hopes to get an impression in the interview situation of how greatly the patient is gifted with real humor, with the capacity for maintaining a sense of proportion as to his place in the tapestry of life. This again pertains more to the personified self than to anything else. There are many things that are called humor by the careless, but I define it quite rigidly as the capacity for maintaining a sense of proportion as to one's importance in the life situations in which one finds oneself.

And lastly, how dearly does the interviewee actually value his life, and how steadfastly, and for how long, has he so valued it? Here I refer to a sense of proportion which is perhaps even broader than the life-saving real sense of humor. What does the person consider to be worth more than himself? For what would he really sacrifice his life? When did that come to be the case? How unalterable is it? How much of it is a matter of mood? As I have said, all of these data bear on a consideration of the personified self of the interviewee, in contrast with all the other data that the interviewer may pick up in an interview.

CHAPTER
VIII

Diagnostic Signs and Patterns
of Mental Disorder, Mild and
Severe

BEFORE GIVING you a list of diagnostic signs—which is anything
but a definitive list—I would like to point out that while almost
every one of these signs can be found in one or another of the
classical mental disorder states, these signs may also appear in
any of us. That is, there is nothing unique about any mental
disorder except its pattern, and perhaps the emphasis laid on
various of its manifestations. Thus we all show everything that
any mental patient shows, except for the pattern, the accents,
and so on.

Diagnostic Signs with Associated Symptoms

The psychiatrist can make diagnostic observations on the
basis of *signs* as they are verified by *symptoms* reported by the
patient. It is well to keep in mind that signs are phenomena
which the psychiatrist can observe more or less objectively,
while symptoms must be reported by the patient; in other
words, only the patient experiences the symptoms. When the
interviewer observes a sign, he must then make certain inquiries
to determine whether there are corresponding symptoms which
are experienced by the interviewee. Otherwise, some facial appearance of the patient's which is genetically determined may
lead the observer into gross errors as to what the prevailing

mood of the patient is. There are some people who have been so heavily accursed by heredity that they cannot avoid looking supercilious. Their expression, however, may not have much relation to the way they feel toward others. When there is a coincidence between what the observer recognizes as signs and what the interviewee experiences, the observer has found an area which warrants further investigation. These diagnostic signs do not mean that the person under consideration has a certain disease, or anything of that kind. They are instead terms fairly rich in useful meaning to the psychiatrist; in other words, they help him orient himself as to what he is up against in the interview and what he has to do. Some of these signs are more apt to appear in the early, more formal phase of the interview, because the patient is not at that time moving with as much self-consciousness as he may be when the psychiatrist really gets down to detailed interrogation. Some signs, on the other hand, are definitely more likely to show up in the more elaborate descriptions of things which take place in the detailed part of the interview.

The first of these signs with associated symptoms is *apathy*. Apathy is a curious state; as nearly as I can discover, it is a way used to survive defeats without material damage, although if it endures too long one is damaged by the passage of time. Apathy seems to me to be a miracle of protection by which personality in utter fiasco rests until it can do something else. An apathetic patient shows no particular interest in the procedure of the psychiatric interview or in anything else. This lack of interest might be described as a certain absence of the presenting aspects of practically any emotion that a person can have. Nothing much in the way of living is going on in such a person. Naturally, many of the interviewer's best efforts to get information prove very disappointing under these circumstances, for the effort of the apathetic person is directed toward simply getting done with things. Of course, if the patient is profoundly apathetic he does nothing; he doesn't talk. But I am referring here to the patient who is just about at the bottom of the ambulatory states of apathy; in such a case the psychiatrist finds that whatever slight response he manages to get is quite clearly an attempt to be civilized rather than any evidence of the patient's feeling that anything can be done in this situation. The patient is simply there, and he goes through certain motions without any expectation of their making sense to the psychiatrist or to himself. Fortunately, we don't see many such people in ordinary times in this country. In certain branches of the military service, and in certain large areas of war-torn countries, there is an excellent opportunity to become acquainted with apathy of all degrees and grades.

Much more common in ordinary experience are states of *sadness* and *depression*. There is just about as much difference between sadness and depression as there is between any two things that pertain to people, but the initial impression does not clearly differentiate them. Depressed people look and sound sad; and if a person looks and sounds sad, the perceived sign is that of sadness. Whether the apparent sadness is a sign of depression—which is a very much more serious and quite different state—will gradually become evident. Sorrow can always be explained. That is, if the person feels willing and free to tell the interviewer what he feels grieved by, the account will be meaningful; there is an adequate explanation for his feeling pretty low in spirit. But the depressed person's explanation for his sadness—if he is able to come out of his depression long enough to make an explanation—puts him in a class with all the great martyrs of history; it is the unpardonable sin, or some such thing, that has brought him down—and this is a mental state somewhat different from sadness. The procedure in interview for these two states is very different. Sadness is quite apt to change during an interview; even a person who has suffered a great bereavement is apt to cheer up somewhat in the process of giving statistical data, and so on. But the psychiatrist who attempts to change depression has a very difficult task.

Practically the opposite of sadness is *elation*, in which one has extraordinarily high spirits. The difference between having extraordinarily high spirits because of a great success, for instance, and being elated, lies in whether or not the person has an adequate explanation for his high spirits. Somewhat in the same direction is *ecstatic absorption*, which an interviewer is seldom able to observe, no matter how skillful he is. In such a state the patient believes that he literally has the ear of God, or indeed that he is a victim of apotheosis so that he has become God. At such times the person is so profoundly occupied with the signal distinctions and the transcendental importance that have descended upon him that he has little time for the mere trifles of living, such as food, drink, income, deference, and so on. *Mercurial change* is a term which describes those who pass in a comparatively short period of time from a lowering to a heightening of mood, without any apparently reasonable basis for the change. Such people can usually be led to manifest these mercurial mood swings during the course of the interview.

Another sign is what I would describe as *overdramatic extravagance* about matters of fact, quite often literally going to the point at which there are no simple adjectives used, but only the comparative or the superlative form of adjectival terms, and so on. The person has had a "wonderful" childhood, a "marvelous" father and mother, and a "perfect" marital partner; he lives a life of the "most beautiful" joy, and so on. Everything is "wonderful." And, since it works both ways, "terrible" things have happened to him too; he had the most "appalling" experience day before yesterday, which may mean, when you come down to earth, that somebody spoke unpleasantly to him. This behavior when it is patterned may characterize what I shall later discuss as hysteria.

Another of these diagnostic signs, that appears even in taking the social history, is *hesitancy* or *indecisiveness*. In such a person the operations seem to be missing by which another person "makes up his mind" and becomes relatively sure that the probability is strongly in favor of one side or the other. To a great many questions such a person replies quite honestly that he doesn't know, that he is not "sure," although he says enough to make another person quite sure. I assure you this is no pose; it is a frightful nuisance to the sufferer; it is no more a pose than the extravagance of many hysteroid people is a pose with them.

The indecisive and the hysterics just live that way—the lilies need a little operation on them before they are quite good enough.

A more positive aspect of this indecisiveness, this doubt as to whether one has gotten the thing straight, is *habitual qualifying*, the routine correction of all statements. A person who qualifies everything he says acts as if no simple statement is sufficient; a few clauses must be added to be sure that there is no misleading of the interviewer. If the latter, in a wise effort to save time, says, "Well, did perhaps so-and-so happen?" with astonishing frequency the answer is, "Well, not quite." After five minutes the interviewer may learn that one of the words which he used wasn't quite the ideal word, and that the patient felt that the interviewer would be misled if he said, "Yes."

The next signs and related symptoms which I would like to mention pertain to the extremely important matter of *tenseness* —that is, the manifestation of tensions which do not seem to be conventionally justified by the situation. One sign of tenseness appears in vocalization. All of us have known from very early in our lives how people sound when they are anxious, when they are tense, in contrast to how they sound when they are perfectly at peace as to their prestige and so on. Without this knowledge we would not do very well in our attempts to communicate. But we may not realize how much we know, and so the interviewer must look for the meaningful changes in tone and so on that occur, in which case he will notice them. Although he probably began to notice such signs in the cradle, perhaps no one has ever talked about them specifically, and so he has no particular frames of reference into which to fit his observations about them. But such frames must be built. Most of the changes in tension during the interview are shown by changes in the voice; even if tension shifts are so gross that anybody could observe them—that is, are shown by bodily movements, by actual blocking, or something of the sort—they are foreshadowed by changes in the voice. In other words, of all our behavior equipment, the voice is probably the most exquisitely sensitive to movements of anxiety. A second, and much more gross, of these signs of tension is tenseness in posture, which, as I have already suggested, is much easier for the inexperienced observer to be certain of. This may show in an abrupt roughness in movement, or in recurrent episodes of real trembling.

Beyond this is what I describe as *gross anxiety*, in which the person shows not only tension, but also various symptoms more or less pertaining to the common pattern of fear, such as sweating even when the room is cold, serious disturbance of vocalization, and general tremor.

A sign which is in quite a different category is what I call *psychopathic fluency*. The patient is very fluent, and seems to have a most estimable past and quite a good future. All of his statements are plausible in their immediate context; they all fit in beautifully with what is being said. With such people the interviewer must be alert not only to changes in the voice, or something of that sort, but also to the improbability that all the things reported by the patient in the course of a fairly long interview could be true of one person. Only when the interviewer raises his eyes from the plausible individual statements to look at the interview as a whole does he realize that astonishingly contradictory statements have been alleged to be equally true of the person. And even when the interviewer questions these fluent contradictory statements, he is unable to bring anything into what I call life relevancy. Instead, everything stays at this plausible, easygoing, conversational level, in which it is very hard for the interviewer to get any test made in terms of "But such and such contradicts this, does it not?" Instead of saying, "Well, I guess it does," the patient provides another burst of plausible utterance—these test situations make no particular impression on him. That is what I mean by psychopathic fluency.

Another group of signs are the *fatigue phenomena*. These are encountered every now and then in many interview situations, and may appear as a gross change during the interview, when the procedure seems to be tiring the patient almost visibly. The phenomena that are of particular concern are loss of perspective as to the relative importance of things, and distinct incapacity to move from one topic to another. For example, the interviewer may have arranged a transition so that anybody should ordinarily be capable of following him easily and be all ready for the new topic; but the fatigued person either is at first somewhat puzzled and mildly annoyed, and then gradually catches up, or he doesn't notice that there has been a transition, and tries to go on with the former topic in some approximation to the interviewer's question. This relative immobility of attention, and the very serious impairment of a sense of the number of things that are important, is striking; in fact, I know of nothing else that is particularly like it. It is important for the interviewer to notice this, because there isn't very much sense in trying to conduct a detailed inquiry of considerable scope when the interviewee is in a state of severe fatigue. The information one gets at such times is almost certain to be seriously misleading, since it will suffer from this relative immobility which restricts the awakening of more important things.

The last two categories in my list of signs, which should have associated symptoms, relate to very much more profound phenomena. The first is *disturbance of verbal communication* with the interviewer, and the second is *disturbance in the gestural components of communication*. By disturbances of verbal communication, I refer to phenomena which no ingenuity of the interviewer can relate directly to felt or avoided anxiety in the interviewee—that is, which cannot be explained on the basis of security operations, in the ordinary sense. The interviewee may have not the faintest notion of what has happened, and certainly has no capacity to realize that he has been made anxious by something.

These phenomena are obscure, puzzling, in some cases bizarre, disturbances of the flow of information by speech. I have sometimes called these the *autistic disturbances*. The term "autistic" pertains to the predecessors of communicative behavior, to the stage of development in which the child has learned something, such as a word, but has not yet attached to it a meaning making it useful for communication. The child may use the

word, may play with it, and may attach private meanings to it
which make it perfectly significant to him, but it is no good for
interpersonal communication. In adulthood, the intrusion into
communicative situations of very private meanings and symbols—autistic phenomena—often has a peculiarly estranging
effect on things. It is not always estranging, simply because we
have all quite probably had considerable experience with this
sort of thing without noticing it. When we do notice it, we feel
rather weirdly at a loss; apparently something has happened
that we don't grasp at all.[1] One sign of an autistic process which

[1] [Editors' note: The text here is taken from a 1945 lecture. In his 1944
lecture on the same topic, Sullivan made the following comments on autistic
phenomena in the interview:

"A commonplace parallel to the appearance of autistic phenomena in the
interview sometimes occurs in the conversation of the people of the Old
South—all of them now very elderly—who still reflect the 'Polysyllabics
Period' in Negro education, as a professor at Fisk once described it. The
state of these people was so unhappy that when they got a chance to learn
something that might be helpful to them, it was a real joy merely to use
words with a lot of syllables. When you converse with one of these old
people, sometimes one of these words, which is tossed in simply to decorate
speech, connects with meaning in your mind; but the meaning doesn't quite
fit the sentence, and so you are a little dashed. And so it is with autistic
phenomena. They appear and they have a somewhat dashing effect. The word
that is used couldn't mean what it ordinarily does; it couldn't describe what
happened.

"Incidentally, let me say here that there are few things more disastrous to
the therapeutic hopes of an interview than for the interviewer to be surprised
at what occurs. Surprise and astonishment on the part of the interviewer are
useful only when forged—when done for effect. When spontaneously expressed, surprise always has a most disconcerting effect on the patient, even
when he was trying to surprise the interviewer; it invariably disturbs the
situation in a markedly unfavorable fashion. Thus when these autistic events
occur, the interviewer should pause a moment before he blurts out, 'What was
that?' For one thing, he may simply have misunderstood. And he might also
consider the possibility that the autistic process was in himself. But if it was
autistic on the part of the patient, that should be carefully confirmed, because it is of very great importance. If there are frequent autistic interferences
in an interview, that almost certainly means that the patient is either in or
near a schizophrenic state. Such people, if they get bad results from one interview because of the interviewer's surprise at what they say, will probably not
return for another interview.

"Thus, without showing astonishment, the interviewer should try to find
out what is really meant. He may be told things which, according to all
ordinary grasp on the universe, could not be so—as in the case of the woman
I have mentioned who said that her breasts were tampered with at night by
her sister who lived a quarter of the way across the United States. In this
particular case, when I asked a further question or two, I found that the

almost anyone can notice, however, is the *absence* of something happening.

First, I might mention what can be described as '*loss of thought*'; the person suffers an ablation, a complete loss of any recollection of what in the world he was talking about; in the midst of something or other, he just draws a blank. Sometimes one is able to discover that a very markedly autistic process swept in and dominated attention, with the result that what was there before is gone really completely. Although such a vanished thought apparently leaves no trace by which it can be recalled, occasionally it can be recaptured by repeating the situation which preceded its loss. A more severe manifestation of much the same thing is 'blocking'; the person is telling something, but then stops suddenly, obviously is somewhat dashed, and by no use of ingenuity can get the topic finished, or take up anything else. He is just sort of stymied, and he is in an extremely distressing, very puzzled mental state in which it looks as if nothing went on, except that he is obviously very uncomfortable about it—and in fact the interviewer is too, usually.

More subtle are *peculiar misunderstandings* or *mistaken interpretations* of the interviewer's questions or remarks, as if autochthonous ideas or actual hallucinations had intruded into the communication. Autochthonous ideas are thoughts which suddenly burst into awareness as if they were terribly important, often as if they had come from "outside" in some fashion. A more spectacular instance of the same thing is the hallucination, in which the person hears, feels, or sees something to which no one else could agree, but the reality of which is not open to any doubt whatsoever by the person who experiences it. As I have said, these things are manifested in the interview situation by peculiar misunderstandings and mistakes—for example, the person may hear something which the interviewer

---

woman meant just what she had said. But it is possible that a patient who made such a statement might, on being asked further about it, go on to say, 'I mean my sister *used* to live out there. She sleeps with me every night now, you see.' Thus it would have been unfortunate to assume immediately that this statement indicated a paranoid delusion."]

has not said, and has not meant to say. Related to these are obscure *emotional disturbances* which the interviewee cannot explain, but which are unquestionably very impressive.

Much less conspicuous, but also falling in this group of disturbances of communication, are *stereotyped verbal expressions* which are simply not communicative. I am not referring here to the people we have all suffered who seem to have a peculiar poverty of expression, so that they use certain hackneyed phrases to cover a great many differences. Some of these people are simply underprivileged, although not all of them are. I am reminded of the young lady whom I admired a great deal when I was a boy; one evening she came along in her sables and jewels with her obviously prosperous escort and looked into the sunset—one of the most moving experiences I believe that many such people ever get on this old globe of ours—and said, after taking a deep breath, "My God, how cute!" I'm not talking about that sort of thing. I'm talking about the situation in which a person uses certain recurrent tags of expression which are not at all simply communicative, they're just things; they obviously mean something to the speaker which they fail to evoke in any way in you. You can find no clue in your experience with the underprivileged or with anyone else that will make these recurrent, stereotyped verbal expressions relevant to the situations in which they are used.

The last of these disturbances in verbal communication is the indication by the interviewee that he feels there are *secret understandings* between you and him, that there is some kind of unknown agreement, that you are with him in some queer kind of unstable conspiracy to ignore certain facts, and so on. He sometimes grows very cute and evasive, and you haven't the ghostliest notion of what he thinks the situation is.

My last grand division of these signs which should be accompanied by symptoms is *disturbances in the gestural aspects of communication.* Here there are three major divisions. The first is *stereotyped gestures;* the person recurrently makes the same movement in the most incongruous situations. You soon come to realize that this gesture is important, even though it often seems peculiarly poorly related to what is going on. It is as if the movement had broken loose completely from any real communicative purpose and instead was serving some very obscure purpose in the interpersonal situation, some end which is very difficult to interpret. The next among these signs are *mannerisms*—peculiar bodily movements which are not the usual accompaniments of certain thoughts and so on. In fact, usually they seem not to have any particular relation to the thought which is being expressed, but go on more or less routinely exterior to the verbal performances of the person, in a quite highly ritualized fashion, so much so that some people have thought that they were automatic and resulted from some irritation in the central nervous system—which is a futile explanation. And last among these disturbances in gestural communication are the *tics*, in which certain groups of muscles seem, as it were, to perform with complete disregard to everything else that's going on. They may range from an extensive contortion of the face, which isn't very strikingly suggestive of behavior, to a momentary start at a smile, a vigorous blinking of one of the eyelids and so on. But in every case they are fragmented communicative gestures, which are apparently grossly unrelated to what is going on. The person is very often unaware of their occurrence, and the only thing that accompanies them as a symptom is that if you can get the person to know when they happen, then you discover that they seem to be more abundant when he feels insecure and so on than when things seem to be going fine. Thus while they usually occur in exceedingly obscure relationship to mental processes, their timing, in particular situations and in the neighborhood of particular topics, may be of some considerable use to the interviewer in directing his attention to certain areas of inquiry.

One difference between tics and stereotyped gestures is that the latter have a much nearer simple connection with meaning, although they are still a fairly long distance away from it. While many people do not know, or only now and then know, when they are showing a tic, they often are aware of, or can easily be led to recognize, their stereotyped gestures, and sometimes they have a pretty good idea of just why they make them at some particular time. More generally, the person doesn't know why he makes a particular gesture, because that is lost in the distance of early childhood; no one at that time told him what it was for, and nobody subsequently has found out. These habitual gestures are rather interesting reliefs, one might say, to various nuisances that one is encountering in living. Sometimes I begin scratching my head, partly because I am sweating, and partly because I am tired; in this way I notice the irritation, and it is pleasant to at least give myself the relief of scratching the place where I am tired. But the way I do it—ah, that's something else again.

Any of these gestural disturbances, particularly when it constitutes a change—when, for example, a tic breaks out in a person who previously has had a comparatively undisturbed facies—may be looked upon as a sort of red flag, indicating that the current topic seems to be of some importance to the person who shows the disturbance.

As I said at the beginning of this discussion almost every one of these diagnostic signs I have mentioned may appear in one of the mental-disorder states, but they may also appear in any of us. Thus the presence of these signs in an interviewee in no sense means that he necessarily has a fully developed mental disorder, either mild or severe. These things appear in everyone now and then, but fortunately they don't always become fixed parts of the person.

But in some people certain processes of living are conspicuously misapplied. In other words, behavior that might be useful for something or other is used by these people to meet problems for which it is singularly ineffective, if not positively the wrong thing. Other people do something that every one of us does at some time during the day, but they do it almost all the time, and thereby seem very eccentric indeed. In such ways disorder patterns are built up from the general repertory of human adaptive performance. Some of these patterns are encountered often enough to get formally named, and the psychiatrist becomes familiar enough with them so that when he sees a part of one of these patterns he expects the rest. He comes to know a good deal about what may be done concerning such patterns and what may have been causal in their formation.

Patterns of Mental Disorder

I shall now present a very brief and quite sketchy outline of some patterns of mental disorder and related personality types. To put this another way, I shall discuss *recurrent eccentricities in interpersonal relations of or pertaining to the so-called mentally deviant, the mentally deficient, and the mentally disordered.*

My first term, the "mentally deviant," is a broad one; if one groups people, in terms of their contact with social reality, their 'intelligence,' or their other characteristics, as the superior, the oh-so-average, and the deficient, both the superior and the deficient may be considered *deviant*. It is important for the interviewer to know whether a particular interviewee is superior, average, or deficient in various respects, but this is not always easy to determine immediately. This difficulty arises in part because the principal medium in the interview is verbal communication, and because of the effect of education on verbal communication. The same difficulty used to arise in trying to determine intelligence quotients: for a good many years, intelligence quotients chiefly measured verbal fluency instead of what they were presumed to measure.

Therefore, it will help the interviewer, in trying to assess the interviewee in terms of whether he is superior, average, or deficient in various respects, to think in terms of a fivefold grouping: the overeducated, the well-educated, the educated, the poorly educated, and the uneducated. He must keep in mind the fact that when he encounters an uneducated person in a single, rather hurried interview, he will have little way of knowing that this person is a superior deviant. And there may not be many clues to the fact that another person is an overeducated mental deficient. Nevertheless, these are important discriminations, because the difference between the outlook of the uneducated superior person and the outlook of the over-educated deficient person is simply enormous.

With these considerations in mind, the first type of deviant I would like to mention—and one which is hard to define very clearly—is the *psychopathic personality*, or, which is the term I prefer, the *sociopath*. Here the interviewer is dealing with factors bearing on the person's habitual contact with reality, which is extraordinarily broad in the superior and extraordinarily restricted in the deficient, and which is intensely restricted, particularly regarding social reality, in the sociopath. In the interview situation, in which the interviewer does not have any too good access to the actual history of the interviewee as many people have seen it, but instead must deal with communication, it is sometimes very difficult indeed to decide whether or not one is dealing with a profound deviation of the sociopathic type, which seems literally to be a matter of incapacity to evaluate matters of interpersonal relations. There are certainly some psychopaths who can realistically read a compass and have just as firm convictions of direction as I have, but what they think of as possible in the realm of interpersonal relations can be looked upon only as fantastic.

I have already mentioned psychopathic fluency as a sign which one may encounter in the interview situation—and which is the sign that suggests to the interviewer that he is dealing with a psychopathic or sociopathic personality. The person is very fluent and plausible in recounting both the glorious and the heartbreaking events of his past. But if the interviewer can shake the facts out of him by any device, it may develop that this glorious past was glorious only in the speed with which he moved from one failure to the next, or took in one victim after another in a sort of witting or unwitting confidence game. And while some of the hard luck stories wring the heart, no one person could have had the remarkable assembly of experiences which he recounts with such convincing fluency. What comes to his mind in a conversational situation is apt to be well adjusted for conversation, but there is no necessary connection between what has happened and what he says about it, any more than there is any necessary connection between what he does and what he very carefully plans to do. Thus his relation with reality is nebulous. Such people have suffered a grave miscarriage of development of personality, occurring after they have become greatly impressed with the utility of speech behavior, with which they almost invariably have a remarkable facility. But while they usually talk very well, they don't realize that some of the things that it is convenient to recall could scarcely have happened if certain others did.

The most difficult problem in deciding whether or not a person is a sociopath lies in distinguishing him from people who are *habitually inadequate and unresisting*—who seem never to rise to any real opportunity, who have no particular capacity to resist any not very useful influence that may bear upon them, and who, like the sociopath, seem to have a restricted habitual contact with social reality. Superficially they are easily confused with the psychopathic or sociopathic personality, but there is at least one rather significant difference: the habitually inadequate and unresisting can, theoretically at least, be benefited by intensive psychotherapy. I have yet to be greatly impressed with that probability in the case of the sociopath.

I now come to a group in which such deficiencies in the contact with reality are only episodic. Among these we find the *epileptics*, and also the people who are what is ordinarily called *'pathologically' addicted* to powerful depressants, hypnotics, narcotics, or other drugs. The lives of these people are strongly colored by utterly inexplicable, or all too painfully explicable, suspensions of their contact with significant events of current reality. With the aid of drugs, the pathologically addicted develop states having some bearing on the characteristic patterns of their life, and very practical bearing on their usefulness for certain types of occupation, and so on.

Next, I would mention *those handicapped by persistent distress or disorder of the somatic physiology*. In this class I would include, first, the *gravely tired*, whose condition is actually tragic, but who sometimes seem comic to others. These people are so profoundly fatigued that they are incapable of those processes which in the more mildly fatigued lead automatically to rectification of the condition. A second subgroup are the *hypothyroid*, who have a deficiency in the endocrine substance secreted by the thyroid gland, as a result of which their capacities for emergency expenditures of energy may be fair, but their capacity for the expenditures required by the routines of life are grossly inadequate. Consequently, these people live in a curiously low key, as it were; even if they do not feel tired, they perform in many connections as if they were. Their difficulty is not fatigue, but a very low metabolic rate, and anything which is beyond that rate, unless it calls out crisis responses elsewhere, doesn't get met. Another group among those handicapped by distress or disorder of the somatic physiology are the *anergic*, without thyroid deficiency. These are the people who have an obscure, but rather grave, deficiency of energy; some of them also have very low blood pressure, although one cannot translate a reading of blood pressure into terms of the energy supply of the person. Many of these people are able to accomplish almost anything in the way of exertion, but are "ruined" when the job is done. In other words, the various emergency resources of the body take care of many things in a sufficiently critical situation, but the general effect—a picture of chronic exhaustion and debilitation year after year—is very conspicuous. The opposite of these, one might say, are the *hypertensive*, who eventually have manifest evidences of the consequences of high blood pressure in the shape of changes in elasticity of the blood vessels—the arteriosclerotic changes—which have a rather profoundly significant effect on the person's living when they involve the blood supply of the central nervous system. So much for those handicapped by conditions effecting disorder of the somatic physiology.

Another major group, which is nearer the realm of the purely psychiatric, is the *demoralized*. While in peacetime such cases are not very conspicuous, in certain disasters of war they are very conspicuous; and they are at all times an important group to recognize. Most people can endure only a certain number of disasters at a certain rate of speed before they pass into a state of demoralization, in which they are practically incapable of initiating anything, although they are able to keep walking, to maintain routines, and to carry on customary tasks. They may not carry these on very intelligently, however.

A somewhat related class are the so-called *deteriorated* people. To illustrate what this means, I shall say that if you were removed from almost all contact with life for five years, with nothing stimulating happening to your mind or your body during that time, and if you were then returned to an active life with others, you would impress other people as being seriously deteriorated. You would have lost touch with the current of life, and unless you were a very remarkable person, or were given much help, you would never regain that touch. In such case you might be said to have "deteriorated" as a result of your experience.

Earlier, in discussing signs which the interviewer may note, I mentioned mercurial change, the sign which suggests the *cyclothymic* type of person. I shall comment briefly here on the cyclothymic people only to give them some place in this outline, and not because I know much about them; I don't. In fact, I suppose I know less about them than about almost any other variety of the human race. These are the people who have profound mood swings; when they are "up" nothing can get them down, and when they are "down" nothing can get them up. When elation (which I also mentioned as a sign) reaches the frankly hypomanic state, the person, even though he may look frightened, acts as if he were feeling fine; he is very gay, and he wants to cheer you up—and now and then he probably pulls some most inopportune wisecracks to do so. It is hard to keep him on the topic long enough to find out anything that carries conviction; and in fact he must get up quite often, and fumble with and admire some of the objects on your desk—and I always feel that next he will have to muss my hair to show how good he feels. It is very much like having the office full of jumping beans. This elated mood is not apt to change during the interview except that it will get worse if you make the patient more anxious. And depression, which looks like a profound state of sadness without an adequate explanation for it, is, as I said before, also very difficult to change in the interview situation.

The behavior of cyclothymic people may be looked upon as an obscure expression of movements away from the experience of anxiety—depression or an unhappy manic state being more tolerable than anxiety itself. The anxiety is apparently rarely felt as such, and it is extraordinarily difficult to isolate the event which threatens to expose the anxiety and in turn sets up the patterns known as manic and depressive. So involved does the observer become in the symptoms and signs, the defensive operations, that the person displaying these remains most remarkably obscure and unknown.

I come finally to a group of mental disorders which are probably of most intense interest to the psychiatrist who is concerned with the theory and practice of psychotherapy. The older nosology in this field is undergoing dissolution, and one may hope that something much better will arise out of the disappearance of ancient errors. I think, however, that the following rubrics still represent important distinctions: (1) those who suffer *anxiety attacks;* (2) the *hysterical;* (3) the *obsessional;* (4) the *hypochondriacal;* (5) the *schizophrenic;* and (6) the *paranoid.* I would like to emphasize again that the people to whom such rubrics refer manifest nothing which is not known in the personal life of each one of you. It is not their manifestations of these processes which is novel, but the misapplication of these processes to things for which they are not particularly suited. It is this which leads to gross embarrassments of others with whom these people are integrated. Thus we come to say that these people are characterized by the misuse of human dynamisms. These characteristic misuses of dynamisms are apt to be relatively durable. There are certain exceptions, however, for they may change under extraordinary stresses. And a frequent instance of change appears in people who have very severe eruptions of schizophrenic processes in lieu of healthy adjustment, for they are likely to move in one of two directions: toward a paranoid development—a misuse of still other processes—or toward the hebephrenic change, which amounts to the deterioration of which I spoke earlier, a shrinking of interest to very primitive, very early levels, separating them strikingly from all the affairs of life.

I shall now discuss each of these rubrics in somewhat more detail. The first of these refers to those people whose outstanding difficulty is their disability by *attacks of anxiety* of the most major character, in which they manifest practically all the symptoms of the most acute fear. These attacks are patterns of fear erupting in interpersonal situations to the point of completely disordering everything except the suffering of the symptoms.

In discussing signs which the interviewer may notice, I mentioned overdramatic extravagance. This is likely to be the sign of the *hysteric*, for it is a rather outstanding trait of the hysteric that no lily is good enough; it must always get a little extra verbal paint. While one may find hysterics who do not show this need to gild everything, when it is conspicuous one may immediately wonder whether or not the person is a hysteric, and by further inquiry can confirm or correct the impression.

Hysterics get themselves disliked with remarkable frequency. For example, occasionally in the pressure of the war I had to work at such high speed that I was not anywhere near par in alertness. I would notice that I was getting terribly annoyed with an interviewee, and begin to wonder what was getting under my skin. Not infrequently I would realize that I had just been listening to one of these conversations in which only superlatives were used, and that I probably had a hysteric before me. One reason why the hysteric is annoying is that the interviewer is quite badly misled for a while if he fails to look beneath the lush, overdramatized, overemphasized picture of things that the hysteric usually presents. Then when the interviewer gradually comes to realize that he has been misled—for hysterics are not so skillful that he can fail indefinitely to recognize it—he is often very angry about it, which is too bad. I think that any interviewee is entitled to be quite skeptical of the skill of a psychiatrist who loses his temper during an interview, or

becomes offended by the patient, for this is a very poor demonstration of skill in handling interpersonal relations. This is quite
different from the psychiatrist's being very unpleasant for a
purpose concerning which he is perfectly clear, in which case
his temper is so sufficiently under control that he can turn it
on and off very precisely for a desired result. Hysterics annoy
me to the point that I realize they are hysterics; in this way my
annoyance can at least be turned to good use.

Another reason why hysterics are disliked is that they are not
uncommonly believed by others to be deliberate malingerers;
for example, they may be accused of being sick for a purpose,
which is really quite stupid of the accusers. At the same time,
there is in the structure of the hysteric pattern a close approximation to what another person would do who was engaged in
deliberate fraud, particularly as to the unfavorable state of his
health. In fact, anybody frequently may do just about what
the hysteric does; this is a peculiarly obvious example of the
fact that these patterns of "mental disorder" are made up of
things which certainly everybody can do, and literally does do
at times.

In this day and age the much more abundant disorder pattern
—which, like the others I have named, is more common as a
marked tendency in this direction than as a disabling mental
disorder—is the *obsessional* state, or, as some people would say,
the *compulsive* state. Obsessional people, when only mildly affected and when employed at types of work which require a
great deal of care about little details, are sometimes really ad-
vantaged by their trouble. The great general principle of the
obsessional state is that the person is so frightfully busy living
that he doesn't have time to suffer some of the greatest pains of
life. Thus, if he can be fearfully concerned about getting every
figure in the ledger precisely correct, and all the sums right, and
so on, going over them eight or nine times so that he then has
the greatest difficulty in catching the bus, he does not have time
to wonder what his wife will throw at him when he gets home.
There is no shadowy vestige of conscious fraud about all this,
and no deliberate purpose in it. In some cases the obsessional

behavior literally penetrates everything, and these people become exhausted with the problem of getting everything right. For example, the obsessional person may develop the most laborious way of putting on a shoe, and the technique may be so elaborate that fatigue, or the dog barking outside, or something of the sort, will cause him to forget one little step, whereupon he must take the cursed shoe off and do it all over again. It may take over forty-five minutes to get a shoe on, and there's nothing funny about that.

If the patient manifests a rather striking predominance of obsessional traits, it is well for the interviewer to be very much aware of this, so that in the earlier interviews he can keep to what he has to know, which is going to be hard enough to do. If, on the other hand, the interviewer, without being aware of the patient's obsessional traits, tries to get anything like a well-rounded picture of him, Heaven help us! he'll be at it forever. It can't be done. We psychiatrists have a flip way of saying, "It's terribly important to the obsessional not to be clear on the most problematic and insecurity-provoking aspects of life," and, if we know what we mean by that, it is so. In other words, when the obsessional person is on the verge of seeing through something that looks pretty disastrous to him, he gets so busy that he doesn't come to see it, and any efforts to lead him to it will, if attempted early in the interview situation, be quite futile, and likely only to lead the interviewer to the grave. Thus it is quite important for the interviewer to spot the signs of obsessional traits in the first interview, and not to wander from the things he must know.

The obsessional states are sometimes related to the schizophrenic conditions by a sort of bridge; and when the bridge isn't there, the relationship is even closer. Such a bridge is composed of a group of troubles which is atrociously named, at the moment, the *psychosomatic* states. The interviewer is not likely to observe signs of the psychosomatic conditions during the recital of social history. However, since they are related to the obsessional and schizophrenic states, if the interviewer in the reconnaissance sees signs of obsessionalism, or encounters autistic interruptions, and so on, it is ordinary common sense for him to inquire about certain parts of the body which are notoriously apt to suffer (be "diseased," as some doctors would put it) as a result of the type of personality problems the person has encountered. Notorious in this field at the moment are the gastric-ulcer syndrome, so called, certain disturbances of lower bowel function, some cases of asthma and hay fever, a few cardiac disorders, and so on. I literally cannot tell you whether certain disturbances of the genital area represent a psychosomatic difficulty or schizophrenia purely and simply. Most surely many of these disturbances in the young are disastrous precipitates of life problems, and often—in part because they are so horribly handled by uninformed physicians, and in part because it is a rather grave business anyway—they represent the earlier signs of severe schizophrenic disturbance.

Thus the field of the psychosomatic disorders should rise to an interviewer's mind when he runs onto a distinctly obsessional person or when he comes across an odd, detached, queer duck —which is, I suppose, the way the schizoid person would ordinarily be described. There is a way of making inquiries about psychosomatic disorders with a minimum of risk. The interviewer may first ask rather casually about the stomach and bowels, as if he were immediately going on to the usually more innocuous subject of the hands and feet. If there is a distinct response, then, of course, the interviewer is interested, but not overly active in pursuing the subject. There are times when you don't try to get a live specimen by setting off a bomb, for to do so might destroy the specimen.

The term *schizophrenia* covers profoundly odd events which are known to most of us only through what happens in our sleep; in our earlier years of life, a great part of our living was schizophrenic, but we have been carefully schooled to forget all that happened then. When a person is driven by the insoluble character of his life situation to have recourse in waking later life to the types of referential operations which characterized his very early life, he is said to be in a schizophrenic state. People who come to be called schizophrenic are remarkably shy, low in their self-esteem, and rather convinced that they are not highly appreciated by others. They are faced by the possibility of panic related to their feelings of inferiority, loneliness, and failure in living. But in all this I see no reason to believe that schizophrenics are startlingly different from anybody else.

The catatonic schizophrenic, who is often mute and engages in practically none of the communication by gesture on which we ordinarily depend, seems to many of us very strange and very inaccessible. However, many years of intense interest have taught me that the patient is rather closely in touch with events, even though for a variety of reasons he cannot communicate. In other words, although there is very little coming out, there are very decidedly things going in. In such situations I proceed with the business of the interview under the restrictions that are imposed by operating with an almost purely hypothetical other person. I am denied what I insist is necessary—any news of who the person is; I must proceed with only the knowledge that he is a person who has a profound disturbance of interpersonal relations which manifests itself in a way that I am by now somewhat familiar with. Because of the extreme handicap on any real interchange with this person, there is a very great possibility of the most serious error in his understanding me, and there is also a strong possibility that a great deal of what I might be inclined to guess or to say to him will be profoundly irrelevant. Therefore, I reduce my attempted communication to certain things which seem to me so very highly probable that the chances of their being irrelevant are small. I then talk slowly and carefully, perhaps saying the same thing several ways, not necessarily in succession, but still trying to cover the ground from various angles. If the patient is "in touch," if I guess correctly what is profoundly important to him at the time, and if I express it in language that is meaningful to him and that connects in his mind with the correct implications, rather than with some very highly autistic content, then I have achieved the objective of the interview. That objective is not primarily my obtaining information, but the patient's receiving some durable benefit. The durable benefit, at this stage, is simply that the patient gets the idea that I am really interested in him, that I take a lot of trouble over him, that I know something about what has probably happened to him, and that I deal with urgent matters of real importance. This is what I have gathered from patients who recovered and later talked about what they recalled of their experience. It was not that after coming out of the dark regions of catatonic stupor they recalled having felt, "That psychiatrist was wonderful! He understood everything!" It was merely that they had gotten the impression that I knew something about what ailed them and that I was interested in them; that was what they needed at that stage, and it meant that they were at least willing to see me again. In other words, if I urgently attempt to keep to those things which are very probably significant, and if I go to a lot of trouble to avoid misunderstanding about what I am trying to communicate, it does have an effect even on these least communicative of people.

It is true, of course, that any psychiatrist who deals with mute patients will find his sense of accomplishment undergoing grave stress. It is very sad indeed to be confronted with fifty minutes of an utterly uncommunicative patient, when you have only one or two ideas that seem to meet the criterion of being highly probable. Long ago I realized that it was not how much time I spent that counted, but the seriousness of my attempt to avoid any possible misunderstanding in communicating what I had to say, and the keenness of my interest in what had happened to the patient. When I have done my best in these respects, and before I am discouraged, I am through, and I leave. It is not useful for the therapist to keep on until he gets annoyed and pushes, for the catatonic can resist this for the rest of time; nor is it useful for the therapist to indicate discouragement and frustration, which the catatonic may recognize as such. I don't believe the catatonic has the feeblest interest in frustrating the psychiatrist; but he has been frustrated so much that he is an expert on frustration. If his psychiatric Statue of Liberty suffers badly from the frustration of his muteness, he may not want to come to America. He may decide it isn't safe. So I suggest that you don't try to continue after you have run out of gas. When you have done your best, depart. It will be no surprise to the patient.

Hypochondriacal preoccupations, as we ordinarily refer to them, shift the sufferer's interest from disturbing aspects of the outer world to gloomy ruminations about the state of his health, impending developments of cancer, and one thing and another *within himself*. Such preoccupations gradually take precedence over all profitable interests in how to pay his income tax, and so on. The hypochondriacal preoccupations, curiously enough, are very apt to skid at times. They are unequal to certain stresses, in which case the patient progresses to the next rubric, the *paranoid state*, in which he makes a massive transfer of blame out of himself onto others. Thus he becomes "blameless" and comfortable, because "not *I*, but *they*" are to blame for those things which are lamentable in his life performances.

CHAPTER
IX

The Termination of the Interview

AN IMPORTANT part of every interview situation is its *termination* or *interruption*. In terminating the interview, or in interrupting it for any length of time, the important thing is to consolidate whatever progress has been made. This progress is represented, not by the interpretations that have been made by the interviewer, but by the degree to which the purpose—the interviewee's expectation of some durable gain from the experience—has been realized. Even if the interview is with a person seeking a job for which he is unqualified, it is the interviewer's business, insofar as he uses the psychiatric method, to see that the person gets something out of the interview. In fact, the interviewer's data are valid only to the extent that he has a lively interest in seeing that the interviewee gets something constructive out of the interview.

The consolidating of the interview's purpose is done, grossly, by the following four steps: (1) the interviewer makes a *final statement* to the interviewee summarizing what he has learned during the course of the interview; (2) the interviewer gives the interviewee a *prescription of action* in which the interviewee is now to engage; (3) the interviewer makes a *final assessment* of the probable effects on the life-course of the interviewee which may reasonably be expected from the statement and prescription; and (4) there is the *formal leave-taking* between the interviewer and the interviewee.

The Final Statement

I don't believe that there is a person in the world who doesn't get something positively constructive from a careful review, by someone who has some judgment of what really does matter in life, of what has been accomplished in, say, an hour and a half's serious interview. Thus the first step in the final termination of an interview or a series of interviews is in the form of a statement; that is, the interviewer makes a succinct survey of what he has learned. As I have suggested elsewhere, this kind of summary statement is useful at various times during an interview or series of interviews. That is, it is useful for the interviewer to repeatedly test the events noted in the interview by stating his impressions of these to the interviewee for his reaction and possible correction. In this final statement, therefore, the interviewer is—insofar as the interview or series of interviews has been successful—stating things which are not open to any ready contradiction or emendation. He is presenting the gross conclusions of which he is by now quite sure. If by chance the interviewee's immediate reaction indicates that these conclusions are inadequate and this seems a valid reaction, the interviewer should take more time and make his summation adequate. But this same reaction may merely relate to the fact that this is a person who must engage in all kinds of hesitating, doubting, qualifying, and so on, in which case the interviewer should merely go ahead as if nothing had happened, having already recognized that it is necessary for this person to qualify everything to the point of uselessness.

In a good many interviews there are things which are heard and inferred about the patient which are not included in the summary. For example, if the interviewer feels that the interviewee has an unfavorable prognosis, he almost never mentions it in a final summary. In other words, the interviewer attempts to avoid destroying what chance the person has. All of these unfavorable things are related to matters which can be summarized, and thus the interviewer can avoid disturbing a patient deeply, and at the same time can review with profit a good deal of what has been observed. For instance, if I were interviewing a person for a highly technical position for which he was unsuited, I would rather carefully omit from the summary any incapacities which seemed to close the door to practically any gainful employment. I might take considerable trouble to emphasize things which made this particular employment potentially undesirable, without, however, making the interviewee feel hopeless or discredited. I have sometimes found it quite useful to propound riddles of this general type to the interviewee who has a poor employment record, a poor study record, and so on: "Well, have you ever thought of a career of such-and-such?"—picking something which seems to be fully as well within his grasp as what he has been considering. Having said something like this, I am inclined to listen, for the interviewee may get started on something. Quite often there is the best reason in the world why such a career is not open to him. But anyway, I may learn more by listening to that than by pointing out all the reasons why he may be a failure. And the patient does not suffer a loss in self-esteem and does not become anxious—and that may be useful for his later progress in other situations. My point is that I try never to close all doors to a person; the person should go away with hope and with an improved grasp on what has been the trouble.

The Prescription of Action

The second step in consolidating the results of the interview is by a prescription of action in which the interviewee is now to engage. The interviewer should offer such a prescription whether he plans a subsequent contact with the interviewee or whether this is presumably his final interview with him.

When the interview is interrupted, however briefly, the prescription which the interviewer offers for the interval is in the nature of homework, as a setting for the next session. For example, I may at the end of an interview mention some point which I am puzzled about because the patient has been unable to recall the details. I may say, "The business of how so-and-so came about is obscure. Well, maybe it will come back to you by next time." In this way, the interviewer can give the patient something to do; whether or not the interviewer suggests home-work, the patient will do some before the next session, and the interviewer may have somewhat better judgment about what might be useful than the patient has.

If the interviewer does not plan to see the interviewee again, he may prescribe that the interviewee is to find someone with whom to do intensive psychotherapy, or, in the case of an em-ployment interview, that he is to look for a kind of job different from the one he came to get, and so on. In other words, the interviewer indicates a course of events in which the inter-viewee might engage and which, in the interviewer's opinion, in view of the data accumulated, would improve his chances of success and satisfaction in life.[1]

[1] [Editors' note: The text here is from a 1945 lecture. In his 1944 lecture on the same topic, Sullivan made the following distinction between the "pre-scription of action" and the usual giving of advice:

"When patients want my advice, I am usually given to some sort of feeble witticism such as, 'Why pick on me? You can ask anybody, anywhere, for advice, and get it. Now why in the world waste your time with a psychia-trist by asking for advice?' If a psychiatrist advises on very adequate grounds, then he is often insulting the intelligence of the person advised. If he advises without grounds, then he is just talking for his own amusement. Therefore, if one is to advise—and certainly the psychiatrist has very often to do this— it is really a clearing of the field for the exercise of foresight, and one usually takes care to do it quite indirectly.

"As I have mentioned earlier, I once gave some advice which was extremely unwelcome, but was perhaps in keeping with an adequate discharge of my professional function. On that occasion I told a psychotic woman that I had no objection to her having a psychosis, which she certainly had in abun-dance, but that if she ever felt like doing anything to any of the 'troublesome' people with whom she worked, I should advise her to go first to Bellevue Hospital. This advice was very harsh indeed, and it promptly terminated the interview; but I think that in that situation I was doing what had to be done. I was saying that the only time at which it becomes really dangerous to have a psychosis is when the behavior may lead to an invasion of the affairs of others in a hostile, punitive fashion. At that time the person is better off in a mental hospital where he is protected from making mistakes.

"Although a person may come to a psychiatrist for help, he may have very real doubts that any such help actually exists. In handling the referral for this kind of patient I may be able to outline the general area and characteristics of some very serious problem with some certainty that the patient can be helped; but I may realize at the same time that the ease or difficulty of his being helped is dependent to some extent upon the skill of the therapist to whom he goes. It is seldom wise to bluntly advise the patient to go to a par-ticular therapist. Instead I formulate the problem as I see it, and discuss the general character of an attack on such a problem and the ways in which a cure could probably be brought about; I then suggest a person who is, to my knowledge, thoroughly familiar with this type of problem and this type of treatment, winding up with a suggestion that an attempt be made to see if this therapist has any free time. When I have done this, I can then strongly advise that the patient get treatment. Thus the advice comes in at the very end to round out the obvious. As a psychiatrist, you see, I sometimes have to round out the obvious because there are people, notoriously obsessionals, who are very unwilling indeed to draw a conclusion—and therefore the psychiatrist gives them the conclusion. Actually, the 'advice' is for the most part an overwhelming display of the factors relevant to the problem, plus a clear statement by the psychiatrist of what he firmly believes can be done about them.

"There are occasions on which one definitely *disadvises*—with force. Occasionally a patient says that he is going to do something, which it is apparent will almost certainly be disastrous. There are several ways of handling this matter, depending on the clarity with which the psychiatrist perceives the irrational character of the act. If it is not clear why the patient is committed to this disastrous course, then I suppose that the way to give advice is to say, 'Why, how did you ever decide upon that?'—and then listen. If the irrational nature of the impulse is quite clear and quite certain disaster lies ahead, it has been my policy to say, 'No!' in quite an emphatic fashion as a way of interrupting the person. I then follow this up by saying, 'Merciful God! Let us consider what will follow that!' Then I try to do that which is really my 'disadvising.' I depict the probable course of events as I expect them to unfold. When I am finished, I turn to the patient and ask, 'Wherein have I done any more than expect the obvious?' If he can show wherein I have been unduly pessimistic, or wrong, I am glad to hear it. If he can't do this, then the situation stands with clear foresight of disaster, and very few people will go ahead with their plans under such circumstances.

"In those cases in which I am not sure that the proposed action is strongly, conspicuously irrational in its motivation, I inquire further, 'Why in the world do you think that?'—with the strong suggestion that I think it's strikingly curious and undesirable. Again I listen. When finally I perceive that the matter is anything but a normal ingredient of a self-furthering plan, I attempt to depict its probable consequences, attempting to call in enough security motives and so on to choke off any direct expression of the impulse. Of course, that does not cure the possibility of irrational acts. I attempt it only when something impends which the patient will clearly regret at his leisure.

"The difficulty which psychiatrists get into by rash advice is often quite simply pathetic. There are few things that I think are so harrowing as the occasional psychiatrist who knows a great deal about right and wrong, how things should be done, what is good taste, and so on and so forth. Such a psychiatrist often feels a missionary spirit so that he wants to pass his own values on to his patients. Not only is this hard on the patient but it also makes things difficult for any other psychiatrist who wants to get something useful done. I think that the psychiatrist's role is to discover the origin of views of indecency and decency, goodness and badness, and so on, except for fields in which there is practically no question. Even when the psychiatrist is quite sure there is no question, it is still always worth while for him to keep a wee crack open in his mind to the possibility of a question existing. I, for example, am bitterly opposed to violence—so opposed, in fact, that I

The Final Assessment

The third step in the termination is the final assessment by the interviewer of what he has told the interviewee in the final survey and prescription of action, and what the effects of this on the life-course of the interviewee are likely to be. In other words, this is a matter of the interviewer's giving some thought to how the interviewee is going to take what he has been offered in this final interview. If the effects of the final statement and prescription of action are not likely to be constructive—if, to take an extreme instance, they have been so discouraging that the patient's prompt self-destruction would be the logical outcome—then there has been some serious deficiency in them, and it is the responsibility of the interviewer to mend this deficiency. As the interviewer grows more skillful, he learns to direct his final statement and prescription of action in such a way that they point to a reasonably constructive picture from the standpoint of the patient. But in any event, the interviewer will do well to assess what this picture is; and if it is not a constructive one, he must realize that he has not yet accomplished his aim—the consolidation of some gain for the interviewee.

The Formal Leave-Taking

There then comes the fourth step, which can really do a good deal of damage if it's done badly—the formal leave-taking. Just as the formal inception of the interview situation is very important, so it is also very important that the interviewer should, as soon as he can, find a way of detaching himself from the interview situation without awkwardness and without prejudic-

try to suppress it in the puppies that grow up around me. Yet there are today on the face of the earth a great many situations in which I recognize that violence is quite the indicated activity. I suppose that years of intense interest in what went on on a particular ward in the mental hospital where I was working has done a good deal to accentuate my intolerance of physical violence around me, for violence on the wards of a mental hospital has far-reaching evil consequences on people other than those directly subjected to it. Yet in spite of my attitude about violence, in general I discourage the practice of giving advice on this subject, or on any ultimate things, great social problems, and so on."]

ing the work that has been done. In actual fact, much good work in psychiatric interviews is horribly garbled or completely destroyed in the last few minutes.

This is just as true of the leave-taking at the end of one interview in a series of interviews as it is of the leave-taking in a situation when the psychiatrist will not see the patient again. As a matter of fact, in dealing with a certain kind of obsessional patient, I have found that the leave-taking for each interview in a series may present a real problem, so much so that for years I have contemplated having two suites of offices. At the end of such interviews, having said my say, I would arise suddenly, step through a door behind my chair, and go to work at my next interview, leaving to the nurse or the secretary the business of escorting my ex-interviewee out, just to avoid the fearful turmoil that such a patient produces in his attempt to get more of something. Just what this 'more of something' is, never becomes really clear to me. These people won't let you be through if they can help it. After you have formulated with the greatest care some really profoundly important truths, and have risen and looked at the door, hoping that the patient will move toward it, such a person may say, "Tell me, Doctor, have we got anywhere today?" or something like that. All of these frantic reachings for some kind of reassurance, or for the Great Formula, have the general effect of confusing all issues that have previously been clarified with so much effort. And so— and I am not attempting to amuse you in the least—the interviewer will be very wise to learn how to rapidly exclude a patient when the interview has come to its end. This takes skill sometimes, but it is very important. In other words, the psychiatrist should not go over things: he should not explain that which is now clearer than it ever will be if he repeats it. The psychiatrist is the expert and he should be expert enough to be done when he is through. Otherwise, much of the benefit of the work can be quite literally wiped out.

So it is in the final leave-taking also. There are ways of getting done with people; and there are ways—it seems to me much more commonly manifested—of having a terrible time disentangling oneself, so that anything accomplished in the final attempt to consolidate the benefits of the interview is confused or exhausted by the efforts of the poor victim and the interviewer to shake each other off. That isn't a good technique. There is no reason why one should have an exhausting turmoil in trying to say good-bye to an interviewee. There should not be all sorts of damnable questions that have long since been answered or never will be answered; there should be a clean-cut, respectful finish that does not confuse that which has been done.

CHAPTER
X

Problems of Communication in the Interview [1]

IN DEALING with people, one must realize that there are always reservations in communication—things that all of us are taught from the cradle onward as dangerous to even think about, much less to communicate freely about. Thus the interviewer recognizes automatically, and as a preliminary to all communication, that no one will be simply 'frank'; such a phenomenon is purely of the language—it does not describe interpersonal relations.

The chief handicap to communication is anxiety. There are times when anxiety on the part of the interviewee is unavoidable or even necessary, but in general an important part of the psychiatrist's work is his use of skill to avoid unnecessary anxiety. There are two important aspects to this "handling" of anxiety: first, one attempts to avoid arousing anxiety; and second, one acts to restrain its development. Reassurance might be termed a third technique for handling anxiety when it refers to a purposive, skillful therapeutic move in interpersonal relations. However, I am not talking here about the use of reassuring verbalisms, which merely represents an attempt by the therapist to do magic with language, and is usually a matter of the thera-

[1] [Editors' note: Unlike the other chapters in this book, this chapter does not represent a lecture as delivered by Sullivan, nor did he include this topic in his outline for his lecture series. This chapter brings together comments which Sullivan made at various times throughout these lectures—sometimes as digressions, sometimes as answers to questions from students—on the problems of communication in the interview, and, in particular, on anxiety considered from a clinical viewpoint.]

pist's reassuring himself rather than the patient. I shall say a few words about this later.

The problems presented in handling anxiety are, it seems to me, vastly clearer if, whatever your initial predilections or previous training, you come to accept my definition of anxiety. As I use the term, anxiety is a sign that one's self-esteem, one's self-regard, is endangered. This is a sign which occurs with a strikingly prospective quality—that is, anxiety is often a sign of *foreseen* lowering of self-esteem. In this sense, anxiety is very smooth-working, and usually not very disturbing, for it usually precedes that which would disturb self-regard, indicating by its appearance that a change must be made in the progression of activity—even if only in the progression of thought—in order to insure the maintenance of an appropriate regard for the self. In other words, anxiety is a signal of danger to self-respect, to one's standing in the eyes of the significant persons present, even if they are only ideal figures from childhood; and this signal, other things being equal, leads to a change in the situation.

In the psychiatric interview, where the therapist is presumably relatively beyond the power of the patient, this change often consists of the patient's doing something to disorder the situation. What he most frequently does, I think, is to become angry, for most people, when even faintly anxious in a relationship with a comparative stranger, get angry, and some do so with their most intimate friends. Next to anger, the most frequent move made to avoid anxiety is to develop "misunderstanding," in which case the person begins talking about something else. This misunderstanding is of such a peculiar nature that I refer to it by the special term "selective inattention," by which I mean that one overlooks, or is inattentive to, that which has provoked anxiety, and shifts to some other topic. If these moves fail, and none of the many others of their kind are effective, the person may experience severe anxiety, in which case he is incapable of any constructive or useful communicative performance.

Perhaps I should comment here on the concept of "resistance" as it may be related to anxiety. Disregarding for our present purpose the derivation of the term and its earlier definitions, I would say that in general it has come to mean *something that opposes what was presumed to be helpful.* I have no great quarrel with the idea that anxiety may be regarded as "resistance." Anxiety is always a handicap to adjustment, and a block to communication, in the therapeutic situation or anywhere else. Any concept that carries, along with its other qualities, some hint that it will reflect unfavorably on the therapist's esteem of the patient will rouse anxiety in the patient and provoke "resistance." That is, following the introduction of the threatening subject, things don't go so well or so simply. The patient begins to use all manner of devices to avoid any four-square collision with the disturbing topic, and the instrumentalities available to the human for doing just this are often exceedingly impressive. But it is of such things as these that the practice of psychiatry is composed. They can be no more than subject matter for further observation and study. They are data.

This sort of thing is not restricted to the psychiatric interview. Even beloved friends—who actually every now and then startle each other by finding out that they have been thinking along the same lines prior to any verbal communication on a given subject—know well that there are some things that one is very careful about communicating to the other; certain things might disturb the other person and possibly threaten the friendship. So it is everywhere. There are always reservations, attempts at clever compromise, smooth evasion, and so on. Thus their appearance in the psychiatric interview is in no sense a reflection on the psychiatrist or his skill; they do not represent the patient's conclusion that the doctor is feeble-minded and can be "taken in." They are necessary, for they are ingrained in the personality. To the extent that the interviewer recognizes them as such, skillfully picking his way between that which is inevitably the case with the patient, and that which is exquisitely adjusted to the interviewer, he can rapidly cut off the illusions of the patient as to what he can get away with, or, to put it another way, what will go unnoticed. If the psychiatrist stumbles in this, regarding as offensive some evasion that is utterly natural to this patient—an evasion that his parents spent a long time engraining in him—the psychiatrist obviously is not an expert in interpersonal relations; his irritation with the patient's evasion miscarries and actually reduces the possibility of a good result.

The first way to "handle" anxiety which I have mentioned is to avoid arousing it unnecessarily, and in the interview this is often a question of progression and transition. Insofar as the work permits, the psychiatrist should try to proceed with simple clarity, so that the patient can follow his direction of thought, for if the patient hasn't any idea of what the psychiatrist is driving at, the psychiatrist, pathetically enough, is not apt to have much of an idea of what the patient means. So it pays, unless there is clear reason for being a bit subtle and obscure, to be quite simply direct and clear. In your personal experience you have no doubt encountered people whose minds leap in such a fashion from topic to topic that every second thing they say astonishes you. With time and enough peace of mind you might figure out how various remarks arose out of what was being said or what had been asked, but by and large you merely have the feeling: "Well, that's a queer kind of person." There are other people to whom it is so very easy to talk that you say a good deal more than you ever intended to say, and if you stop to consider why, you will usually find that each topic grew "naturally" out of that which preceded. Or if events did not proceed in the most "natural" way, then there was very probably a quite careful attention to transitions, so that you were never surprised. The questions which were asked seemed to be the right, sensible ones, and the other person seemed always to show a rather sensitive comprehension of what you were attempting to evoke in his mind; and so it was very easy to go on and on.

In the same way, the competent interviewer usually introduces each new topic with certain conversational gestures which conclude the current subject and open the mind to something new. If he presents a new point of view or a difference of opinion, he does it in such a way as to clearly indicate that there is no reflection on the interviewee's standing as a personality. Any patient who comes to a psychiatrist is apt to be insecure, and this insecurity will considerably increase whenever the patient must stop and think, "Now what is the doctor getting at? What does this lead to?" Such an increase in insecurity is almost certain to play a good deal of hob with the interview.

I would like to say a few words here about "blocking." This is a term of rather indeterminate meaning, but commonly refers to a state in which the progression of approaching speech through awareness—the preparation of things to say—is very seriously disturbed by contradictory impulses, one of which does not predominate. In other words, the impulses have practically equal importance, as a result of which the patient says nothing, and feels very awkward. He is not likely to be aware of the contradictory impulses; at some point of "disagreement" or "misunderstanding," he simply draws a blank.

Most of the things that we say are reviewed before they are spoken. This is a very swift process, for there is a great deal to be reviewed. A person who is reasonably sure of what he is attempting to do, and reasonably sure that a very large number of errors and inaccuracies are bound to happen, will often say things which need to be modified after having been said. That is, even as he passes from the initial review, which is extremely hurried, to hearing it as the other person has heard it, he realizes that it is inadequate and in need of correction. If all of this procedure is blocked at the moment that one gets ready to speak, it is easy to understand why very little comes to be said.

The extent to which a person will be free of blocking is to a large degree the result of the ease and freedom with which he can say what occurs to him, and so the simple and easy progression of inquiry will often avoid the precipitation of blocking. For example, asking a direct question will sometimes result in a kind of blocking. However, you may not even notice it, for we have all, in the process of growing up, become skillful at accommodating to what amounts to a lack of communication with the person with whom we are talking; and so you may assume that something has been communicated which has not. The indirect question, composed of running comment, additions, corrections, and so on, which imply what you want to know, or suggest the information desired, is possibly the ideal way of getting information in such a way that you can be reasonably certain of what is being communicated.

Thus, in general, it is wise to avoid disconcerting cessations of communication, and to proceed by steps that are within the grasp of the other person, so that he feels that he knows what you're driving at, and therefore knows what he's talking about. This is what I have earlier referred to as the "smooth transition" in the interview.

A consideration that may lead to your *not* being so simple and obvious in the train of your questioning is again that of avoiding arousing anxiety—that is, guarding against any unnecessary discomposure of the patient. There are some areas in the inquiry in which you do not permit the patient to follow your thought—when it is desirable for the patient to be, as it were, out of touch for a moment, in order to avoid his having too troublesome a train of thought. You don't plunge gaily into things that are going to make him horribly tense and uncertain as to how you will respond to what he says. Furthermore, when the intervention of anxiety makes it impossible for the patient to go any further in a particular direction—when you see that his tension is increasing to the point of interfering with communication—you will find it wise to move emphatically out of the particular topic which is being discussed into another. Perhaps you can come back to it later. As a matter of fact, most topics of human living are so interlocked that you can approach the same thing from six or seven different directions. It sometimes happens that something which provoked considerable anxiety when it first came up is much less intimidating to the patient when it is later investigated from another approach. Because people are often unable to communicate anything when they get very anxious, you should not go out of your way to discompose a patient unnecessarily—in fact, you can show your skill by avoiding that.

I make one of these emphatic moves out of one topic into another—"abrupt transitions," as I call them—when I foresee that there will not be, in the particular interview, enough time to get the patient's anxiety down to reasonable proportions. Certainly, in the earlier stages of psychiatric work, it is very risky to let a person get intensely anxious and then cut off the interview because the clock has gotten to a certain point; that is a way of intimidating patients on the whole subject of psychotherapy, which may delay almost intolerably their really getting deeply to work—and it is also a way of increasing the rate of suicides and admissions to mental hospitals. One of the heaviest responsibilities of the psychotherapist is to try to get the patient on the downgrade of anxiety before the end of a session, instead of in a state where he is becoming increasingly anxious. When the patient's anxiety is mounting, this abrupt transition, in which you simply rip apart the communicative situation and present another—where there is a sudden change of topic at your behest—usually comes as a very distinct relief to the patient, and it can have a distinct educative influence also. For example, in the earlier phases of the interview, before what I would call a dependable situation has been established, if I see a patient getting pretty tense about something in the last part of the session, I often turn around to face him fully, or in some other way indicate alertness, and say, "You're getting quite anxious, aren't you? Well, what's the hurry about this? We can drop it and go on about so-and-so, can't we?" Now, that is what I would call a very abrupt transition. The educative element is in what I say about anxiety; I want the patient to understand why I broke in, but I don't want to give him a dissertation.

Incidentally, dissertations—these fine, windy explanations by the analyst of what he is doing and what he thinks, and so on—are very, very apt to miscarry in the earlier stages of the detailed inquiry; some of my colleagues have worked with very gifted analysts, but heard almost nothing that the analysts said to them for the first year or two. They knew it was terribly important, but somehow they just didn't quite follow it—it didn't leave much of any trace. I think the development of psychiatric skill consists in very considerable measure of doing a lot with very little—making a rather precise move which has a high probability of achieving what you're attempting to achieve, with a minimum of time and words. If you realize the importance of the transitional effect in a communicative situation, you will find that you can spare the patient extensive discourses, which in the early stages of psychotherapy almost never communicate what you suppose you've said, even though you may say it beautifully. Often the patient doesn't hear any of it; an authority is speaking, and he feels that all he has to do is maintain an attitude of reverence and be ready to do something when the authority stops.

Another grave limitation to the smooth and easy progression of inquiry appears when you have become so involved with the patient's self-system that you are being sold an extended piece of goods—that is, being misinformed by the minute, which is very expensive to the patient. In this case, an easy progression of inquiry will merely keep up an unfortunate motion. I use an accented transition to suppress these security operations. I may not change the subject, but I do change the communication by showing traces—or sometimes very glaring amounts—of satire, boredom, restlessness, annoyance, or something of the sort. Now, I don't recommend that to others; each psychotherapist brings to his work his own equipment which he uses every day with other people, some of it for good and some for ill. The problem for every psychotherapist is to sort out the things he does well with others and try to build up his psychotherapeutic armament out of those.

So far, I have been discussing chiefly the techniques of progression and transition in the interview as ways to avoid arousing anxiety and to restrain its development. Incidentally, it is the latter problem which most people have in mind when they say, "How do you *handle* anxiety?" In other words, they are not referring to anxiety as a rather smooth-working advance warning of danger to one's self-esteem, but to the very severe loss of euphoria when the person feels that his security actually *has* diminished, when his self-regard, or his estimate of another person's regard for him, actually is greatly reduced. When the interviewee suffers such a gross loss of euphoria, it is sometimes possible for the interviewer, moving very swiftly after the signs of anxiety appear, to restrain its development by some means other than transition, or sometimes to reassure the patient—provided, as I said before, this is not merely a matter of using reassuring verbalisms. For instance, sometimes the interviewer may ask a question which leads the interviewee to make what he feels is a most damaging admission, so that he then becomes intensely anxious—although he may cover the anxiety by equally intense feelings of anger or other emotion. The remedy lies in the interviewer's then asking a question about the "damaging admission"; for example, he may ask, "Well, am I supposed to think very badly of you because of that?" Now this may seem like a strange kind of operation, but its value is that it puts into words the content of the interviewee's signs of anxiety. The answer is ordinarily "Yes," and the next step is to ask, "Well, how come? What is so lamentable about such a thing?" Without waiting for an answer, the interviewer explains that while the interviewee may regard the event concerned as something to be greatly ashamed of, and so on, such happenings are quite the universal experience of human beings; while the informant may not know this, the interviewer can scarcely avoid knowing it, and so he is not very much impressed with this "damaging" data. That completes that process. The interviewer can then inquire where in the world the interviewee got the impression that this particular thing which has caused anxiety is so deplorable. In all of this, if the interviewer moves smoothly, naturally, and in a manner unstudied enough to carry conviction—instead of giving the impression of merely being very clever in the technical sense—he may discover something of real importance in the person, a vulnerability in the organization of the self which is especially related to some particularly pestilential moral censure in the past.

The reassurance of schizophrenic adolescents seems to consist almost entirely of this sort of thing—trying to discover just what in the world is supposed to be so terrible, and what in the world is terrible about it. One thing that used to be terrible in male adolescence was masturbation; I don't know how it is now, but in my earlier years this "practice," as it was called, carried a heavy load of moral censure. Sometimes when I was interviewing a male adolescent I would say, after prodding around for a while and drawing blanks, "Well, I suppose you're another of the people who has been ruined by masturbation. Is that it?" The patient often would nod to indicate that such was the dreary truth. I think that my asking this question was usually in itself extremely reassuring to the patient, for it introduced the idea that many people regarded themselves as ruined by masturbation, but that I had other views about this matter. Having thus created the impression that this was by no means the first time that I had heard this sad and somewhat erroneous story, I would say, "Now tell me, how much did you masturbate to accomplish this ruin?"—I would endeavor to get across some faint satire by this repetition of "ruin." I would usually find that the person masturbated once in a fortnight, or something like that, and then I would want to know how long this had been going on. And as I prodded away at this topic, I would seem to be struggling against an all-encompassing boredom, and that too was often reassuring, for it showed that I was not at all excited about this supposedly terrible business. After I had found that the young man had had a frightful struggle for the past two and a half years, swearing off repeatedly, only to fall back into the miserable habit, or something of the sort, I would rouse myself from almost a stupor, and say, "Yes, I see. Now tell me, how did the ruin appear? How did things begin to go wrong?" At this I would begin to get an account of his relationships with people, and I would get more and more interested as that went on. Perhaps an hour later I would say, "Now why is it you connect masturbation with all this? How do they get mixed up together in your mind?" If by that time I had been successful, the person was apt to say, "Well, aren't they connected?" I would say, "Yes, by the fact that you experienced all of these things, but I don't know how otherwise." With this I might feel that I had done a fairly good job.

The point is that there is no use trying to reassure an adolescent—or anyone else—if you don't know what you are reassuring him about. And you ordinarily don't know what to reassure him about, aside from a few good bets such as masturbation used to be—and even in that case, you still had to be told about it before you could do anything about it. You cannot do magic with reassuring language. The magic occurs in the interpersonal relations, and the real magic is done by the patient, not by the therapist. The therapist's skill and art lie in keeping things simple enough so that something can happen; in other words, he clears the field for favorable change, and then tries to avoid getting in the way of its development.

Some patients show the ways in which they are distressingly insecure by displaying a marked need for reassurance. For example, upon being asked in the reconnaissance if he married his first love, a patient may hesitantly reply that he didn't, and then begin to wonder if that is all right. He wants to be told whether he should or should not have married his first love; there is almost a clutching for agreement that he is all right, that he may go on living, that there is nothing to be ashamed of. All of this grinds up a lot of time. Yet the insecurity which the patient is showing is a very important aspect of his problem, and something that is quite worth finding out about.

Some such people try to make a hash of everything without knowing it by groping for some magical reassurance at the end of the interview. This may happen at the end of a first interview, with a patient you are undertaking to treat, or one whom you are sending to someone else for treatment; or it may occur during the course of intensive psychotherapy. In any case, you should not attempt any private miracles at the end of the interview. There is no justification other than your own insecurity —which is no justification at all from the patient's standpoint— for any attempt to reassure unless you are in a position to document what you say. I am not suggesting that the interviewer should curtly throw out the person who suddenly says at the end of the interview, "Tell me, Doctor, have we gotten anywhere?" But in this situation I do try by my response to make

the patient aware of the extreme irrelevance of his final performance, and yet leave him integrated enough to be able to
think over the interview. Thus I may look at him with surprise
and chagrin and mutter to myself, "For God's sake!"—and let
him make what he can of that; I hope to invite his attention to
the preposterous nature of his attempt to pull that kind of a
rabbit out of the bag.

Some interviewers, particularly those who are inexperienced,
feel called upon to pour some healing balm on the victim at the
finish of an interview, as if finding out what the trouble is were
not in itself a life-size job. Such therapists tell a patient that although they are not quite clear on what the trouble is, they are
very sure that they can find out what it is, and that it can be
fixed—which, so far as I am concerned, is utterly gratuitous
magic. In fact, it may disturb the patient when he thinks it over,
for I don't believe that it is particularly good for a patient to
realize how much distance has yet to be covered before the expert knows much of anything about what is going on.

Occasionally a patient asks fairly urgently at the last moment
if he can see the doctor on the next day, looking as if he were
having violent anxiety, and were preparing to do something
about it. My suggestion in such a case is to indicate a time on the
next day when the patient can call to find out if you have time
for a session. There will probably be a lucid interval, perhaps
when he is on his way home, or when he is going to bed that
night, during which he can take stock of what has happened.
If, after this stock-taking, he still wants to see you next day, he
can always call up and find out if it is possible. But if he actually
feels greatly reassured as a result of the lucid interval, and you
have already agreed to his request, he may feel somewhat like a
fool; and, incidentally, since it is unpleasant to feel like a fool,
he may wonder whether you, the expert, may not be a bit of a
fool too, or whether you have nothing to do except run in emergency appointments next day.

All in all, when you can't reassure a person except by magic,
the sensible thing is not to try. When you don't know anything
in particular to say, don't say it. Yet you need not resort to curt

refusals when the patient wants reassurance at the end of an interview. Instead, you need only realize that the interview, so far as you are concerned, is done; and so far as the patient is concerned, the phase which is perhaps most important is only about to begin—the retrospective appraisal of what he has undergone. Try to leave things so that that will happen, because it can be very valuable.

I mentioned earlier that a common manifestation of anxiety is talking about everything but the problem. Then, people sometimes ask, how do you find out what the problem is, and how do you get the person to talk about it? The rule, so far as I can formulate one at the moment, is this: If you know how you arrived at the point at which anxiety put in its appearance, you can often guess what seemed to be ahead from the standpoint of the interviewee. If you follow closely what is discussed, trying to promote easy communication and to keep things moving, you will observe the patient veering off from certain topics in a fashion which strongly suggests the general area of the problem. If you approach this area, you notice that the patient more or less skillfully shifts to talking about something else before arriving at it. But notice that the failure to arrive after just *one* approach doesn't prove anything beyond the simple fact that you didn't arrive; in such a case you do not know wherein the difficulty lies. However, if you try two or three times, coming in from rather different angles toward much the same topic, each time without success, you are then in a position to say quite simply, "I notice that you haven't had anything to say about so-and-so. Obviously it is difficult to discuss it." And putting the obvious into words often markedly improves things. Then the patient can say with considerable force, "Yes! I don't like to talk about that." Then I can be amazed, and my amazement means, "Well! I don't see that that follows at all. What's so difficult about it? How come you dislike it? Is it supposed not to be respectable or something?"

I would now like to mention a communicative situation which arises when the patient loses some of his caution, exerts less effort to maintain distance from the interviewer, and feels more free to say what is in his mind. He will then begin to experience more keenly the significant people of his past. There will be times when the patient will so distort the psychiatrist because of the situation that has been revived in the patient that a *parataxic situation* exists. In such a situation there are actually three people: the *'imaginary' psychiatrist* to whom the patient is addressing his behavior and words; the *patient* who is reacting to this 'imaginary' third person; and the *psychiatrist* who is observing and trying to get some clue as to what this imago to whom the patient is reacting might be like. If the psychiatrist identifies this role and fits it long enough to become a perfectly convincing illusion or delusion to the patient, he is in a position to inquire of the patient, "Is it possible that you think I am actually thus and so?" Whereupon the patient may say, "Why, of course." The psychiatrist can then say, "When did you begin to think that?" Having discovered when all this began, the psychiatrist says, "But isn't this curious? You recall that I said so-and-so and several other things that are incongruent with this imaginary person." The patient may say, "Yes, it is curious." At this point, the psychiatrist says, "Well, now, tell me—there must have been someone in your past, very significant indeed, who acted like that. Who occurs to you?" Whereupon the psychiatrist may discover who the really significant person was in the patient's past—that is, the person with whom the patient has been in an inferior position, whether the relationship was one of tenderness or otherwise.

Such intrusions of past people do not appear until after the patient begins to feel safe in saying various things to the interviewer which ordinarily he would not say. After that point is reached, the wise interviewer notices whether things begin to be a little bit strange in some way or other; he tries to learn what this strangeness consists of by inquiring about it, and thereby learns about certain people in the patient's past, the great significance of whom may never have been clear to the patient.

A special instance of the avoidance of anxiety is found in the problem of relating to the paranoid person in the interview.

The anxiety of the paranoid person is intensified by any impulse to draw close to another person. If anything occurs which makes the paranoid person feel that someone is being kind to him, is loving to him, wants to make him feel friendly, and so on, he experiences anxiety. As he experiences it, this anxiety is a sign, a warning, that he has overlooked something, and that the "friendly" person is endangering him. Therefore he usually reacts hostilely, although his reaction may be delayed. In many cases the therapist discovers that because he has been quite nice to a paranoid person, this person is put to the necessity of inventing a more or less delusional idea of what the therapist is trying to put over on him.

Thus it becomes almost a first principle for the therapist to be distant in dealing with paranoid people. He may, in fact, often be rather forbidding. I am sure that I have received a great deal of information from some paranoid people because they felt I was a thoroughly disagreeable person. I asked unpleasant questions unpleasantly—and got some answers. If I had asked unpleasant questions in a friendly way, these people would probably have gotten all tied up in knots about what I was trying to get at, and what I was trying to convict them of. But when all that they ordinarily supplied to a social situation—unpleasantness—was provided by me, there was no danger of their feeling friendly toward me, and therefore becoming anxious and suspicious.

Thus, while the therapist ordinarily should try to make things run rather smoothly, with the paranoid person he should go to some trouble to make all implications, especially the unpleasant ones, very clear. For instance, I have suggested that, in dealing with the adolescent schizophrenic, it is very useful if the conversation proceeds so smoothly from here to there that the person feels amazingly comfortable and gets to talking about things he had no intention of talking about, and so on. But with the paranoid person—to take the same sort of instance I have just discussed—if I say, "Oh! and I suppose you figure that masturbation destroys you, eh?" I make it sound very cold and almost insulting. That is the trick, for if he feels that I am possibly a little bit tough, the greatest problem a paranoid person has—people who act "friendly" toward him—does not arise. Such people give him a feeling of acute disadvantage. That is what anxiety is; it is a warning of impending disadvantage, and immediately calls out suspicions and various "righting movements."

Unless the proper precautions are taken—and with experience the taking of these becomes almost automatic—the interviewer may get involved in some very serious delusional misinterpretation. There is a way of handling such a misadventure. If you have a certain mental agility and a clarity of focus on what is currently happening, you can put into words the nature of the misinterpretation, saying something like, "Do I understand that such-and-such is the case?" The patient may say, somewhat guardedly, "Yes." Then you say, "And pray, out of what was that built?" You then review all the data which may have been twisted to fit into such a picture. As you hit on a particular event that was woven into it, the patient usually gives some sort of sign—an increase of muscular tension or something of the sort—and then you rather sardonically tear up the suspicious character of that innocent event. In this way you rip up the whole thing piece by piece. And you can wind up with some semblance of being outraged at having your time wasted by such misinterpretations. You may find that *he* is outraged at the discovery that you have "shown him up." You must overlook that; and the only way that you can do this is by seeming to be annoyed at how things have been misinterpreted. Then, as a final move, you say, "And how often do you suppose that kind of misunderstanding comes up in your ordinary life?" That question makes sense. The problem is no longer localized in the relationship of you and the patient. You have suddenly become a competent psychiatrist; you have uncovered his difficulty, and have verified the natural history of a particular instance of it. At this the patient will usually mutter something like, "Well, it's possible that it happens now and then"—whereupon it's my practice, however unpleasant, to say, "Yes, I surmise at least that frequently," and we are on our way again.

If I seem to be suggesting that you insult paranoids, I have failed to make my meaning clear. I don't know what would happen if you insulted such people; the results might be exciting. But in any event don't, for the sake of all concerned, try to befriend them. I *do* know what happens then, and it is exciting, but very unpleasant. What is important in these relationships is to maintain distance, a rather unkind, but actually very careful, reserve. By that locution, "unkind but very careful," I mean that you administer no wounds that do not heal. Taking falls out of people is no part of the psychiatric interview, unless it is necessary to open the mind to something that must be dealt with. The interviewer can be quite unpleasant, if he is sure that he isn't unpleasant at a point, or in a way, that leaves an open wound. Anything which makes a person feel "small," if you please—a really excellent figure of speech—is apt to leave a long-enduring wound, and to be anything but a help in the further development of the interview. The interviewer tries very carefully not to belittle or humiliate people; he can be remarkably unpleasant and distant, without actually humiliating in any way other than by interpretation. Humiliation or belittling that requires interpretation before it is experienced may be interpreted in retrospect in a different way, and thus is not so lastingly hurtful.

I hope I have made it clear that the psychiatrist should avoid giving tacit consent to delusion or to very serious errors on the part of the patient. Let us say that you are a young psychiatrist, and that the scion of a very wealthy family, who has been referred to you for treatment, comes in and tells you something, the probability of which impresses you as being very near nil. It may seem the most natural thing in the world to say, "Oh, yes, yes! Is that so?"—and to go on with something else. But you pay for such things at your leisure, and gradually learn to do better, because the patient in such cases doesn't stay with you a very long time. The patient probably doesn't stay very long, either, with the psychiatrist who brashly and firmly asserts, "I can't believe it!"

In these cases, you should first confirm, by asking the most natural questions that would follow, that the patient intended to say what he did, and that there was no misunderstanding on your part. Having made sure that the patient's statement was as bad as it sounded—that he is entertaining an idea which is not only wrong, but also, in a sense, does violence to the possibility of his living in a social situation among others—you do not then say, "Oh, yes, yes. How interesting!" You rather say, "I can scarcely believe it. What on earth gives you that impression?" You note a marked exception.

That is all you need to do, in my experience, in order to go on with the interview. If something seems terribly off the beam, you register your amazement and ask about it; even if you don't get much information, at least you note your exception, and do not agree tacitly. Often I merely shake my head as if it were just a bit beyond me, conveying a rather strong negation. The patient is often quite grateful that I am not willing to go along at once with a marked misapprehension about something; although he may not be able to say it to me directly at the time, he, too, would like to get rid of these troublesome distortions. Always remember that no matter how sick a person is, the chances are that he is still more like you than he is different.

Curiously enough, the fact that the psychiatrist doesn't start a holy war about the patient's delusions, but at the same time isn't agreeing with them, often gives the patient the impression that the psychiatrist may be sane and is not in any plot against him—and therefore something may come of it. If, however, the psychiatrist says, "Oh, yes, yes. Very interesting. And now tell me about so-and-so," changing the subject, the patient may get the idea that the psychiatrist is a fool, poorly trained, or part of a plot—no one of which ideas is particularly helpful to therapeutic progress.

I wish now to comment on a rather commonly asked question: What is it that brings about favorable change in a person? How do patterns of living undergo significant alteration for the better?

The thing that keeps people from favorable change, from profitable return on certain of their experiences, is that they do not learn anything from those experiences, or, if they learn anything, it is not enough to produce much benefit. It may be surmised that something specifically stands in the way of such learning. But if one assumes that man is as highly adaptive as I always try to suggest that he is, the great question is: Why does a given person not overcome the handicap to learning? Why is he not moving forward? The answer lies in the fact that at some time in his past it became dangerous for him to inquire into certain aspects of what happened to him. That is, such inquiry became so fraught with anxiety that he goes on year after year feeling threatened by experience in some particular field. That experience may be anything from telling a superior what he really thinks about something, to approaching apparently genial members of the other sex with an idea of perfecting his acquaintance with them by genital behavior. Whatever it is, he has been taught by early experience to shy off, to permit no tests, to make no adventures in this dangerous field. When the field concerns lust, or some other very powerful motive, he may make ventures in it, but only after surrounding them with such precautions that they are practically useless.

An example of such precautions is provided by the person who is quite promiscuous but never has sexual relations except when seriously intoxicated. Incidentally, it has been very well stated by some one of my colleagues that alcohol is that material by which one tests the ideals of a personality, ideals being notoriously soluble in alcohol. The sort of person I am describing is afraid to do certain things, and yet is seriously driven by his motivational system to do them; thus he has hit upon the happy idea of so divesting himself of his more complex capacities that he can engage in this behavior with considerable vagueness as to whether it was *his* wish to do so, or *somebody else's*, whether it *did* or *did not* happen, and so on. Under these circumstances, unhappily, experience is very seriously garbled by the impairment of the person's ability to maintain clear contact with the environment.

What I am driving at is this: When a person comes to an interviewer with a problem, the assumption is that this person has been *restrained from using the totality of his abilities*. The problem of the psychiatrist in treatment is to discover what the *handicaps* to the use of his abilities are. I believe that this is quite profoundly and generally true. Let me illustrate as follows.

After certain oddly confusing motions by a patient which I have learned usually mean that a "Great Problem" is about to be revealed, and considerable delay at which I finally show some slight impatience, he may say: "Well, I have a sexual problem." Since I suspect that at this rate we'll get nowhere in an hour and a half, I may say, "And doubtless a homosexual problem." The patient then says, "Yes, Doctor, that's it." Then I may learn that my patient has often had sexual relations with a member of his own sex, or that he has been unable to think of having relations with a member of the other sex, or *something*. That's what this "homosexual problem" means to me—just "something." The *real* problem which I hope finally to uncover, to my patient's satisfaction and with his clear insight, is *what stands in the way* of his making the conventional, and therefore the comparatively simple, adjustment which is regarded as normal. In other words, I don't treat any alleged entities such as homosexuality. I have come to recognize homosexuality as a developmental mistake, dictated by the culture as substitutive behavior in those instances in which the person cannot do what is the simplest thing to do. Thus I try to find out why he *can't* do the simplest thing, and in such investigation may come to solve the problem.

Consider again the question: By what dynamisms does one change? Invariably one changes by the removal of obstacles to perceiving where one is and what the situation that confronts one is, and why it has been so difficult to perceive these things. In some ways that is the great problem of the interview itself: what is the patient's situation, how can the interviewer discover it, and to what extent can the patient accompany the interviewer in discovering it? Thus when you encounter a person with a "homosexual problem" (in quotation marks, for homosexual is only a name), what counts is what you discover about the person—what particular terrors, menaces, and risks other people hold for him. Quite often that leads you back into the very early years of his life, and through their study change comes about. In problems which bear upon such important things as relative security with members of one's own or the opposite sex, change cannot be brought about in a few interviews. Nor will change occur quickly when the problem reflects years of effort on the part of the parents to indicate to the person that he is unable to get along by himself. There are a great many other things that cannot be changed quickly, simply because the anxiety which the patient undergoes in presenting the relevant facts is so great, and because nothing can be learned by him until that anxiety is lessened. In other words, a person must feel fairly safe in order to make use of anywhere near 100 per cent of his abilities. If he feels extremely insecure, he will be unable to present adequately the simplest proposition, and unable to benefit from its discussion.

Thus we try to proceed along the general lines of getting some notion of what stands in the way of successful living for the person, quite certain that if we can clear away the obstacles, everything else will take care of itself. So true is that, that in well over twenty-five years—aside from my forgotten mistakes in the first few of them—I have never found myself called upon to "cure" anybody. The patients took care of that, once I had done the necessary brush-clearing, and so on. It is almost uncanny how things fade out of the picture when their *raison d'être* is revealed. The brute fact is that man is so extraordinarily adaptive that, given any chance of making a reasonably adequate analysis of the situation, he is quite likely to stumble into a series of experiments which will gradually approximate more successful living.

Sometimes a patient asks: "Doctor, how can I do better at what it is vital to me to do?" And sometimes a therapist asks: "What do I do to be of help in all this?" The answer to both questions is this: work toward uncovering those factors which are concerned in the person's recurrent mistakes, and which lead to his taking ineffective and inappropriate action. There is no necessity to do more.

Conclusion

WHAT I HAVE said in these lectures is intended to pertain to the practical work of interviewing in the psychiatric manner, which was defined as that type of relationship with the interviewee that would produce dependable data on something important about him and bring him benefit. That is what makes it "psychiatric," you might say, in contradistinction to all the other types of cross-examination, and what not, to which people are subjected.

You may feel that all this has been very impractical, in that you could not possibly in the next five or ten years get to the point of covering all that has been touched on in this very sketchy, skeletonized outline. My aim has not been to be pleasant and discursive, or provocative, but to present schemes for organizing one's thought, outlines of approaches, and the type of data that would be relevant in such approaches. I do this with two things in mind: first, that you will get an idea of the general framework that must exist in the psychiatric interview, and an idea of practical ways of setting up this minimal framework; and second, that you will then devise the outlines, schematizations, and so on, best suited to you, which will encompass the essential data and make best use of the interview time. I have given you not a definitive plan, not a carefully thoroughgoing detailed outline of any particular phase or aspect of the interview, but a suggestion of what the outstandingly significant data are.

Until an interviewer has opened his mind to the rather intimidating complexity of interpersonal relations and of those hypothetical things, "personalities," which enter into them, and until he has organized a rather systematic way of keeping all these data in mind, he invariably overlooks a great many events. This is all the more so since all conversation between two people is directed by attempts to avoid insecurity on the part of both of those engaged in the verbal intercourse. Many of the people whom the interviewer sees have developed quite subtle ways of maintaining security, and unless he has a fairly organized notion of what are likely to be the relevant data and how extensive they may be, and has a great many schematizations handy in his mind, he may be led into blind and unprofitable alleys, and may be very successfully deflected from important areas by the unwitting skill of his interviewee. It is for that reason, chiefly, that it has seemed to me important to present, not a definitive statement in each of these fields, which I could never adequately formulate, but a large number of the high spots characteristic of each. Let me say very simply that I never expect anybody to have all the information about any interviewee that I have suggested as being obtainable and important. For instance, if one is interviewing someone fourteen years of age for the position of office boy, with a view to his emptying wastebaskets before the office force arrives, and seeing that there is ink in the inkwells, and so on, it is not really profoundly important that one know his outlook toward life. As a matter of fact, I would expect the outlook toward life of a fourteen-year-old to be quite a transitional phenomenon, subject to remarkable changes in the course of his employment in any stable office. Thus there are many things that may have no particularly high relevance to a certain situation. But it is nevertheless important that we, as interviewers, have a rather clear idea of what is significant or not in the behavior of humans. It is, at least in part, through our ability to observe events and to evaluate their significance in the life of the interviewee that we may come to serve some useful purpose to him.

Throughout this discussion of the interview situation, the interviewer has been considered as an expert in interpersonal relations. That is, the interviewer is alert to interpersonal phenomena not only in terms of the interviewee's behavior but also in terms of what happens in his own behavior and in his covert processes. He is careful in dealing with the interviewee's anxiety as evidenced in multiple reservations and attempts at deception. He checks adequately any important parataxic distortions which seem to be present. He notes where information seems to be lacking and in some cases supplies it. And finally, he never ignores the limitations of his own experience and the restrictions which are imposed upon him by his role as an expert in the observation and interpretation of interpersonal phenomena.

The course of the interview situation proceeds on the basic assumption that the interviewee can derive at least some durable benefit from his contact with expert skill, but that this can occur only in the measure that a valid relationship comes into being. Thus the interviewer must handle himself like an expert in interpersonal relations from his first meeting with the patient, through every detail of the formal inception of the desired situation, through the reconnaissance into the social identity of the client, through the detailed inquiry into all that is highly relevant to the success of the interview, and finally in the carefully organized termination or interruption of the contact. In this expert role, the interviewer is seriously interested in the problem presented by the interviewee; he is careful to avoid misunderstandings and unintentional erroneous impressions; he is ready to be corrected, yet chary of repetitive, circumstantial, or inconsequential details; he foregoes the satisfaction of any curiosity about matters into which there is no clear technical need to inquire; he eschews all procedure chiefly calculated to impress the client with the interviewer's clairvoyance or omniscience; he avoids all impractical meaningless comment, the clouding of issues, or tacit consent to dangerous delusion or error that will be difficult or embarrassing subsequently in the interview; he proceeds in general with such simple clarity that the interviewee can follow the direction of the inquiry; and from time to time, he offers his impressions for correction or discussion by the interviewee. And finally, the interviewer as an expert makes sure that the interviewee 'knows himself' the better for the experience.

Index

Addiction, *see* Narcotics, use of
Adolescence, 137–138, 150–152, 214–216
Advice in the interview, 201n–202n
Alcohol, use of, 154–156, 224
Allport, G. W., 68n
Ambition, 146
Anergia, 188
Anger, 103, 127, 207
Anxiety, 94–95, 128–129, 224–226
  attacks of, 190, 191
  gross, as diagnostic sign, 178
  as problem in communication, 206–221
  See also Self-system
Apathy, 174–175
Attitudes, 144–146, 152–157, 170–171
  cultural, 9–11
  in interview situation, 75, 107–108, 112–115, 120–121
Autistic, the, 143, 179–181
Autochthonous ideas, 181–182
Awareness in interviewing, 64–65
  See also Participant observation

Blocking, 181, 210–211

Case material, 20–22, 23–24, 86–87
Catatonia, 195–196
Change in patient, 107–115, 116–121, 223–226
Childhood, 96–97, 134–135, 139–142
Chronology, 60
  written, 84–85
  See also Reconnaissance, the
Communication, 116–119
  anxiety in, 206–221
  disturbance in, 179–184
  nature of, in interview, 5–9
Competition, 144, 145–146
Compromise, 144, 145–146
Compulsive states, *see* Obsessional states
Conceptions of Modern Psychiatry, Sullivan, 75n
Covert processes, 54–55, 92
Culture:
  attitudes of, 9–11
  handicaps of, 34–35
Current data, 163–164n
Cyclothymia, 189–190
Data, use of, in interview, 29–32, 51–55, 138–172

collateral, 58–63
  See also Reconnaissance, the
Delusions, 221–222
Demoralization, 188–189
Depression, 175, 189–190
Detailed inquiry in interview, 38, 77–78, 212–213
  developmental history as frame of reference in, 130–172
  as a process, 107–129
  theoretical setting of, 89–106
Deterioration, 189, 191
Developmental eras, 132–138
  See also Adolescence; Childhood; Infancy; Juvenile Era; Preadolescence
Deviant, mental, 185–186
Diagnostic interviewing, 40–41
Diagnostic signs, 173–185
  See also Mental disorder, patterns of
Dissociation, 125–126
Dynamism, 125–126

Eating habits, 157–158
Education, data on, 71–72, 185
  formal, 135
  See also Schooling
Elation, 175–176, 189–190
Employment, data on, 60, 71–72, 163–165
Epilepsy, 187
Euphoria, 96–97
Expert, role of psychiatrist as, 11–12, 26–34, 63
Eyes, delusion about, 5–6n

Family, data on, 69–74
Fatigue, 178–179, 187–188
Free association, 77, 78–80
Frustration, 125–126

Games, 144–145
  See also Recreational activities, data on
Gesture, 179, 182–184

Hallucination, 181–182
Hebephrenia, *see* Deterioration
"Here and now," 28
Hesitancy, as diagnostic sign, 176–177
Homosexuality, 86–87, 225–226
Humor, sense of, 172
Hypertension, 188

231